INTRODUCTION

Obesity is a global epidemic; that much is certain. Put simply; obesity is a condition in which your body has too much fat or has way more fat than is healthy or convenient for it. Apart from being a physical disturbance and discomfort, obesity poses some serious health problems that are often hard to manage and sometimes even harder to prevent. Compared to people with normal weight, people living with obesity are generally considered to be at risk of developing certain diseases. The abnormal medical conditions that obese people are predisposed to coming up with include, but are not limited to, diabetes, hypertension (persistent high blood pressure), high LDL ('bad') cholesterol or low levels of HDL ('good') cholesterol, heart diseases (including coronary heart disease and cardiac arrest), stroke, diseases of the gallbladder, sleeping and breathing abnormalities, certain types of cancer, bodily pains, psychological problems (such as depression, anxiety, and some other psychological abnormalities), and generally low quality of life. It is worthy of note to state that not all people who are obese go on to develop these health problems in the course of their lives, but equally noteworthy is the fact that obesity makes you more liable to come across these and other health challenges. The risks are simply higher for people embodying more fat than they should.

A person is said to be obese when their body mass index (BMI) is found to be above 30 kg/m^2. The body mass index is obtained by dividing an individual's weight by the square of their height. Although the threshold for full-blown obesity has been pegged at 30 kg/m^2, a person who has a body mass index in the range $25 - 30 \text{ kg/m}^2$ is considered overweight. Obesity has been a major global health challenge for a long time now and, although there have been countless services and products rolled into the market to help counter the trend, the epidemic has seemingly ignored all of the countermeasures and become more rampant over time. Unlike most of the world's health epidemics that are caused by disease-causing pathogens, obesity is caused mainly by any combination of excess food ingestion, physical inactivity, and genetic makeup. Apart from the obesity cases caused by the aforementioned factors, there are a few other cases that have been reported to arise as a result of intake of certain medications, endocrine gland abnormalities, and some mental health conditions.

Some people living with obesity have been wrongfully led to believe that there is little they can do about their condition, and perhaps due to their frail state of mental health (which sometimes accompanies obesity), they accepted it as true. This belief leads them to indulge more and more in the behaviors that caused the obesity itself, and the downward spiral goes on from there. Contrary to this false notion, there are a number of effective measures you can take to shed excessive fat. These measures include exercise, dieting, surgery, and fasting. Of all these, fasting is considered by many as not only the most cost-effective and least stressful option but also the easiest to accomplish and sustain. Fasting for weight loss is approached in the form of intermittent fasting, where you cycle or alternate between periods of eating and not eating, hence the term 'intermittent.' Unlike dieting which takes into cognizance the calories you ingest and tries to regulate what you eat and how much of it you take, intermittent fasting does not place restrictions on the kinds of food you can eat. Rather, it places emphasis on when you eat. Intermittent works to help you lose weight in a healthy manner, simplify your life, improve your overall health condition, and reduce the effects of aging.

Intermittent fasting counters the leading causes of obesity, such as overeating, eating too often, and genetics by cutting down the sheer amount of food you eat and the length of time that you eat for. During normal and fasting days, your body makes use of the muscle glucose that comes from the food you eat for its energy needs. When the glucose levels in the muscles are depleted, the body fashions a means of converting its fat into a useful form of energy to continue to carry out its metabolic activities. This process leads to a decrease in the amount of body fat and a consequent loss of weight.

Intermittent fasting assists your weight loss endeavor by making you eat less and for shorter periods of the day than what you would consider normal. Through several fasting regimens, you can channel your weight loss efforts through healthy pathways and achieve the weight and life that you want. There are many intermittent fasting protocols to choose from, which would be presented in this text. However, there is room for flexibility in the fasting options; you can literally take a fasting protocol and modify it to suit your unique needs and capabilities. You could even combine a number of fasting protocols and alternate between them till you achieve the weight you are genuinely comfortable with. The options are seemingly endless.

Unfortunately, many people do not really understand the rave about intermittent fasting and why so many people seem to be joining its bandwagon. That is not surprising as intermittent fasting is not as definitive a diet as other common weight-loss diets. Rather, it is more of an eating plan than a diet.

I have written this book to help clarify the grey areas that come in play when you decide to join the intermittent fasting family. Why should you take up fasting? How does it fight weight loss and other ailments?

Naturally, I will proffer more reasons within the book, but to sum it all up, intermittent fasting is the true, natural eating plan that humans subscribed to a long time ago. It follows our roots that we do not eat every time like herbivores. Yet, unfortunately, most of us have turned the plan upside down. These days, we all eat ourselves to a seeming stupor each time we catch sight of any food around.

Unfortunately, our body system has not been designed with appropriate checks to deal with this large influx of food of all varieties and quality. This leads to a major impasse when it comes to gut and overall health. In the same way you will expect sludge to build up in an engine that is not properly maintained, our body soon begins to slow down too. It may start from a loss of control over eating periods or present as eating disorders, but the true way back to true sanity is intermittent fasting. With time, this loss of balance begins to affect biochemical processes as well, and that is the basis upon which metabolic diseases and conditions such as obesity, stroke, gut inflammation, and general ill-health develop upon.

Intermittent fasting eliminates physiological imbalance and provides other psychological benefits. This book discusses the nitty-gritty of fasting including plans, rules, and its potential demerits. Intermittent fasting is a better, healthier way of eating and living, and you do not want to get left behind.

CHAPTER 1

BENEFITS OF INTERMITTENT FASTING: HOW INTERMITTENT FASTING IS THE BEST WAY TO SOLVE WEIGHT LOSS ISSUES

If you are a skeptic, you may think that intermittent fasting may just be one of those overhyped dietary trends around. Quite truly, fasting is not new; it has been in existence for as long as humans have lived. Until the last few decades, the human species has had a period of no eating. Fasting has over time been incorporated into our culture and diet and can yield a lot of benefits to our bodies and minds, both at a physical level and on a molecular level, something we are only just starting to understand and appreciate.

We are fortunate enough to be in abundance of food provisions in this era, but this was not always the case in our history. Some of our ancestors and predecessors didn't have enough food to feed on. Intermittent fasting, quite frankly, has its roots in ancient times. Our ancestors were hunters who went out to seek and hunt games, which they gathered in the night times for feasting. When they did come home with food, they would make fires and roast their hunts. When the hunt did not go according to their plans, however, they usually went hungry and famished. Therefore, because of these feasting and fasting alternations, the body systems of our ancestors learned early on to adapt to the circumstances. Hence, it was normal for a person in the ancient world to go days, weeks, and even months without much food to eat. These times that passed without adequate food to eat made our bodies go through *hormetic* stress, which later turned into something beneficial to us. When there is an absence or insufficiency of calories, our bodies tend to activate protective genes that are geared up to provide for cellular repair and protection duties in order to sustain life. In addition, these genes are also responsible for preventing inflammation or reducing it to a bare minimum and improving the body's defense mechanisms against oxidative stress. Therefore, going on without food for some time can guard against inflammation, aging, tumors, and many other chronic abnormalities of the body.

Intermittent fasting is markedly different from every other eating pattern and practice. It is not a diet *per se* as it does not focus on eating a particular group of foods or avoiding others. Instead, it focuses on promoting healthy eating by limiting either the time you can eat or the amount of food you can consume indirectly.

Fasting has always been present in various religions and customs since time immemorial. So, it is pretty much natural for humans. However, and also, it is our natural mode of eating. For instance, Ancient man would eat when food was available and then carry on his activities until he felt famished again. He didn't store food; so, he begins to search for food only when he is already hungry. That constituted a fast in between when he got hungry, and when he could find food to quench his hunger. Our ancestors underwent daily fasts that helped him to keep his metabolism and weight in order. It is part of why they lived much healthier lives full of vigor and natural existence.

In our time and day though. Things have changed. No one needs to search for food before he eats. Every minute of the day, we have food thrust in our faces and mouth. Ads, jingles, and brazen display of cooking ensures that hunger is no longer an effective biological measure for remaining in shape. Instead, everyone everywhere seems to be eating our way out of shape and into a stupor. In fact, "unhealthy eating habits" appears to be the real, new fad. The vast majority of people have numerous destructive eating habits that pose a threat to their health, yet, only a few recognize this. From this few, only a microscopic number take proactive measures to curtail these habits. Many pick up underlying nutrition patterns that they give up soonest because they cannot cope with the requirements. Therefore, a very tiny proportion of the entire population of the world has healthy eating habits, even though many want to.

The solution is not as far as portended. The answer is to return to our nutritional roots by way of intermittent fasting. Luckily for you and me, intermittent fasting can get you back to as natural a shape as possible by teaching us new healthy habits.

Intermittent fasting is rooted in the belief that you can lose weight by eating better. The methods of accomplishing intermittent fasting for the sake of weight loss are deemed some of the safest weight-loss strategies and have been used extensively to not only lose weight but also to help improve general body health. In the right doses, intermittent fasting can achieve health wonders in a relatively short period of time. Some of the proven benefits of intermittent fasting are as follows:

- **Weight loss:** Weight loss is perhaps the most popular benefit of intermittent fasting and one that most people who indulge in intermittent fasting seek. Intermittent fasting is thought to provoke weight loss by decreasing insulin levels in the body. When we eat carbohydrates, the body breaks it down into glucose (which is the smallest functional unit of carbohydrates). It is this glucose that the body cells use to produce their energy by further breaking it down. Under normal circumstances, not all of the glucose produced is used by cells to produce energy; the excess glucose is converted into fat and stored by the cells for later use. During this process, the hormone insulin promotes the intake of glucose by the cells. However, when a person is not ingesting food, insulin levels decrease. When a person fasts, the body's insulin levels are dropped, forcing the cells to utilize the glucose reserves, including those stored up in the fat cells. This process, when repeated over and over again, has a capacity to reduce body weight. Additionally, intermittent fasting makes you consume fewer calories in general, which may lead directly to a reduction in weight.

  The major factor that guarantees weight loss in intermittent fasting s the regulation of the amount of time your system spends in the 'fasting' and 'feasting' states. When you just finish taking a meal, your body enters into a feasting state during which, for about three hours, it attempts to digest and thereafter absorb the food nutrients you had just eaten. In this state, a lot of calorie-burning activities takes place, and energy is produced in abundance. Following this period is the fasting state, which your body lunges into in the absence of food to digest. Depending on the particular intermittent fasting protocol you are on, the fasting state could last for up to twelve hours at a stretch, and during this period your body, low on glucose, begins to use up the glycogen in fat deposits to produce the energy it needs to carry out its activities. Because we seldom go for twelve hours on end without eating, very few people are open to utilizing this fat burning process. This is the major reason why intermittent fasting can achieve huge results in the area of weight loss in a relatively short period of time, and that too without putting you through the agony of having to make some other lifestyle modifications.

To support the assertion of the weight loss potential of intermittent fasting, an academic review published in 2017 in the journal of Molecular and Cellular Endocrinology took and assessed data from 40 different scientific studies on intermittent fasting. The authors of the study came to the conclusion that intermittent fasting is useful for weight loss. It is useful to point out that intermittent fasting has a similar level of effectiveness as traditional calorie restriction diets and is being considered by many as the easier option.

- **Intermittent fasting can control blood sugar and lower your risk of developing type 2 diabetes:** The body's fuel of choice for carrying out its everyday activities is glucose. Glucose is a product that is obtained from the breakdown of carbohydrates or starchy foods, such as bread, rice, and potato. Ingested starchy foods get broken down into smaller, absorbable units, glucose, in the gut from where it is shipped into the bloodstream. Whilst in the blood, insulin, the primary hormone that works on glucose, gets the glucose from the blood into the body cells that utilize this glucose to satisfy their routine energy needs. This is to say, for cells to have the energy they need to perform their activities effectively, there must be insulin present, and it must be active and effective. Sometimes the cells get so much glucose that they can't possibly take much more; in this situation, the excess glucose is stored as glycogen in fat and liver.

As you continue to eat, excess glucose continues to pile up and continues to get pushed into fat deposits in the body. These deposits of glycogen can lead to weight gain when stored in body parts such as the abdomen and thigh. During fasting, the sheer amount of sugar that needs to be acted upon by insulin is reduced, and this leads to a consequent reduction in the amount of glycogen pushed into the liver and fat deposits. This goes a long way in reducing the amount of work that your insulin has to do and can optimize its performance.

When you fast, the body falls short on glucose. This lack of glucose forces the body to search other places for its energy needs. The body sources energy from certain other substances, an example of which is ketones. When there is a shortfall of glucose, the body resorts to burning some fat for energy. Fat deposits all over the body are stimulated and burned to meet the energy requirements of the cells and, in the process, ketones are produced. These ketones, mainly acetate, acetoacetate, and beta hydroxyl-butyric acid, are generated from the burning of fats and used for energy purposes. This process of generating energy from ketones as opposed to from glucose is known as ketosis and is triggered when you are fasting.

According to the Obesity Society, nearly 90% of people living with diabetes type 2 are either overweight or obese. Therefore, losing some weight helps in the management of this type of diabetes, as has been proved over and over again in studies and clinical trials. Weight loss is effective in the treatment process of type 2 diabetes because it helps the body to reduce insulin resistance and makes it able to absorb glucose better. The major cause of type 2 diabetes is a development of resistance to insulin, a situation where the cells, muscles, and certain organs find it difficult to absorb blood glucose. This situation leads to above normal levels of glucose in the blood, a condition known as hyperglycemia. Drugs that can reduce the body's resistance to insulin are usually recommended for people with this type of diabetes.

Type 2 diabetes is the commonest type of diabetes in humans. It is the type of diabetes that reduces the body's capacity to produce insulin, a hormone needed to break down the carbohydrate into glucose and which controls blood sugar levels. It is thought that intermittent fasting can have a positive effect on the prevention of type 2 diabetes. Obesity is one of the commonest risk factors for type 2 diabetes; intermittent fasting releases fat and helps you lose weight, thereby improving your body mass index. This directly reduces your risk of developing type 2 diabetes. While routine calorie restriction diets can help reduce weight and lead to a similar level of reduction in insulin resistance, intermittent fasting goes a step deeper by reducing serum insulin, which stimulates the body to use up stored sugar (glycogen) together with fat when there is an absence of glucose in ingested food. The processes of burning stored sugar and fat are thought to have a capacity to reduce sugar levels in the blood and trigger weight loss.

A 2014 review article published in the journal of Translational Research assessed all current evidence that intermittent fasting can reduce the risk for developing type 2 diabetes by lowering the blood levels of insulin and glucose. The researchers concluded that intermittent fasting done correctly can effectively lead to weight reduction and a decrease in the risk of developing diabetes.

- **Improvement in heart health:** Intermittent fasting has also been found to have positive effects on certain areas of heart health. It has been linked to a reduction in blood pressure, heart rate, cholesterol level. Even though researchers are yet to know exactly why it is observed that intermittent fasting has the potential to decrease the risk factors for developing heart disease. It is also in theory that individuals who have a fasting diet are apt to have better heart health than those who don't. This is perhaps due to the fact that people who fast have a stronger grip on what they eat and how many calories of foods and drinks they consume. The improved eating habits of such people can translate directly to a better state of heart health. While a decrease in the risk factors associated with heart abnormalities is an enormous feat on its own, routine dietary fasting can also have an effect on how your body acts of sugar and cholesterol.

- **Intermittent fasting could improve mental health:** Although it has not been proven in humans, intermittent fasting is said to have a positive effect on mice's learning and memory potential. This bodes well for humans on intermittent fasting regimens, as they can be sure of reaping similar rewards. It is also theorized that intermittent fasting has the capacity to improve brain health by preventing inflammatory processes from taking off. Intermittent fasting also improves cognitive function, at least in the lab mice that experiments have been conducted on. During fasting, a certain protein that resides in nerve cells, called the brain-derived neurotrophic factor, BDNF, is produced. This protein has an important role to play in learning, memory, and the production of fresh nerve cells in the brain. This factor also strengthens nerve cells, making them more resistant to stress. In addition, fasting also stimulates the process of autophagy, in which certain cells get rid of destroyed or damaged chemical substances and inhibit cell growth.

  Therefore, during fasting, nerve cells seem to be in a mode that is primarily focused on conserving resources and resisting stress. Once you eat after you have fasted for a while, cells make a shift from the resource conservation mode to a growth mode in which they produce tons of proteins and grow. These alternating periods of resource conservation and growth may play a significant role in improving learning, memory, and resistance of the brain to stress.

- **Possible reduction of the risk of developing cancer:** Intermittent fasting can reduce the risk of developing certain types of cancer, according to scientific studies conducted on mice. Certain studies on mice have concluded that intermittent fasting and some other restrictive diets can reduce the risk of cancer formation. However, no studies have been conducted to link intermittent fasting with cancer prevention in humans. Despite the dearth of studies linking it to cancer prevention in humans, you can rest assured that intermittent fasting is likely to head in that direction. This assertion is true because it is already proven that intermittent fasting has reducing actions on insulin level and inflammation. Insulin level and inflammation both have links to cancer.

- **Intermittent fasting contributes to several positive processes in the body:** Several processes are kick-started in the body during fasting. When you fast, your body initiates a number of processes directed toward repairing damaged cells and alters the blood hormone levels to make stored fat more useful. In addition to these:
  - Body fat is actively burned as insulin levels decrease.
  - The levels of the human growth hormone increase significantly, up to five times the normal value. When blood contains these high levels of the hormone, a perfect environment for fat loss and muscle gain is created.
  - Intermittent fasting also plays a role in gene expression, where it makes positive changes to what genes are expressed by repaired cells.

- o   Autophagy is another process that is triggered in the body during fasting. It is a process whereby the body repairs damaged cells and tissues and generates new ones. This means that when you fast, you are literally letting your body carry out some overdue repair work.

- **Reduction of oxidative stress and inflammatory reaction:** Oxidative stress is a condition that sets in as a person ages. It deals with certain unstable chemical substances known as free radicals that react with some other chemical substances in the body (including proteins and DNA), damaging them in the process. Intermittent fasting can improve the body's defenses against oxidative stress. Furthermore, intermittent fasting can help prevent inflammation, which is another major cause of chronic diseases.

- **Intermittent fasting may be useful in preventing Alzheimer's disease:** Alzheimer's diseases is one of the commonest degenerative diseases of the brain in the world today. As there is currently no medical cure for the disease, preventing it from even developing is crucial. It is theorized that intermittent fasting can help prolong the onset of Alzheimer's disease or reduce how severely it affects the brain, as studies on mice show that it is promising in achieving such. In addition, intermittent fasting has been shown in animal studies to help prevent Parkinson's and Huntington's diseases. Although more research in humans a=is needed to arrive at any reasonable conclusion, these studies show a spark of what intermittent fasting could achieve in the area of neurodegenerative diseases.

- **Prolongs lifespan:** Intermittent fasting has also been linked with an increase in the lifespan of humans. This is coming off studies conducted on animals that showed that intermittent fasting increased the lifespan of rats much in the same manner as a persistent calorie restriction regimen does. It is no surprise that intermittent fasting can achieve this feat, as it has already been proven to help improve several metabolic processes and reduce the risks for certain inflammatory disorders.

- **Promotes conscious, healthy eating habits**
Discipline is a big part of healthy eating. The development and maintenance of a healthy eating habit will have a significant advantage in our lifetime. Being conscious of one's intake does not only lower the risk of cancer, heart disease, diabetes, and other illness, it also makes you feel healthy and look better. Conscious and straightforward effort can be made for you to adopt some changes in your diet and make healthy eating a natural way of living life. The tips you are to take towards attaining this include;

Cultivating the habit of regular breakfast goes a long way in elongating a healthy lifetime. It supplies your daily nutritional requirement, regulates your blood sugar level, and gives you energy. Foods you can consider for breakfast include; Yoghurt topped with fresh berries and granola, peanut butter, cottage cheese with fresh fruit, whole-grain toast, and cottage cheese

Consider planting a garden at your backyard and fill it with decorative outdoor planters. You can make use of fruit and vegetable plants such as cherry tomatoes and strawberries. Fruits that have beautiful color add a kind beauty to the garden. By the time you start to harvest the beautiful, nutritious, and new things you have earlier planted. You will be encouraged to consume them and thereby promoting a healthy eating habit. You have to be conscious of your mealtime as well. Try getting a suitable place, and avoid any disturbance while eating so that you won't encounter any emotional stress or unnecessary argument that will later result in a digestive problem. Eat at a reasonable pace, not too fast, and stop eating when you observe you are satisfied. One of the healthy way to about with your eight management is knowing your body's satisfaction signal.

- **Reduces the volume of food eaten**
When it comes down to it, everyone likes an extra scoop of ice cream or another plate of an omelet. Wanting food is no crime, and neither is overeating. However, reducing your intake is not to say that you should subject yourself to hunger. All you need to do is to ensure there is a reasonable reduction in the amount of food consumed daily

One of the steps you can take is the consumption of more protein; it gives you a kind of fullness and makes you take less while having your next meal. This helps you lose unnecessary fat without undergoing hunger. The intake of protein helps you prevent muscle loss and reduces daily calories.

You can as well go for foods that are rich in fiber, this stretches the stomach and slows down the pace at which it gets empty and this, in turn, releases the hormones. Reasonable drinking of water can go a long way in reducing the amount of food you take in a day. It decreases the level of hunger you feel before taking the meal. Research has made it known that individuals who take two glasses of water just before their meal consumes lesser food than people who do not take water prior before eating their meal. For people that love to takes things like ice cream and the likes. I suggest you go for chocolates, preferably dark chocolate. Although it is bitter, it helps to decrease appetite and reduces the rate at which you crave for sweets.

Ensure you spice up your meal, the capsaicin present in hot peppers and sweet peppers helps to step up the feelings of being full and thereby reduces hunger. Getting a regular exercise will reduce your appetite by going by the fact that it makes use of your stored fat as the source of energy. Research has made it known that the level of neuronal reaction to food decreases when you undergo moderate to high-intensity workouts.

Getting an exercise as well reduces the incentive present in the brain which is responsible for hunger. It minimizes the anticipation for food, reduces stress, and make you healthy. Lastly, various research has been made on getting enough sleep and otherwise. To cut a long story short, not getting enough sleep increases the hunger hormones, which later result in the large volume of food intake. So getting enough sleep is a way to stem the food intake.

- **Gets rid of junk**
Although junk can be addictive, there is a specific moment in which you will be salivating for junk. If you happen to fall in this category, you are not alone, so many other people crave for this frequently. It is a known fact that manufacturers ignite a kind of addiction. They ensure consumers get their utility as the junk are produced in such a way that the

sweet, salty, and flavors are at the moderate level. However, having talked about addiction, it is important to talk about possible control to it.

The first step to go about this is to ensure you get a proper plan ahead of your mealtime. An already planned healthy meal for your lunch will most likely prevent you from going for Pizza, French fries and sweets. Try shopping at the typical section when you get to the grocery store, ignore where junk is packed and shop where you get real dairy, fish, vegetables, grains, proteins, and grains. Add more delicious food to your routine. Once you start enjoying the various diet, you tend to forget about the intake of junks. A perfect example is adding a new green to your salad, or get a specific type of fish.

The moment you start negatively thinking about junks food, the lesser you crave for it. A research that was made on people trained to think negatively about junk shows how quick their orientation changed about it. Some already got full and tired about it. Some sneezed immediately they set their eyes on it, some felt it could be saved for later. Generally, the negative consequence such as weight gain and stomach ache was revealed.

- **No diet restrictions, so no risk of deficiencies**
  Making good sure that you eat a balanced diet is key. When there is no restriction of a certain class of food, it's indicating that you will most likely not be affected by any deficiency. Dieting itself triggers overeating in some situation. Take this for an example: if you do not take brownies, immediately you see it with someone turns your sensor. Also, the restriction of food groups such as sugar makes one feel deprived and can lead to overeating.

CHAPTER 2

PROTOCOLS OF INTERMITTENT FASTING: WHAT ARE THESE PROTOCOLS, AND HOW DO THEY WORK?

People have utilized many different protocols of intermittent fasting to achieve their various fasting goals. While some have employed calorie-restricting measures, others have resorted to using the time restriction technique. However, whatever the pathway you choose to follow, the result will be most likely the same. Some of the most common protocols of intermittent fasting are the 16/8 protocol (also known as the lean gains method), the 5:2 protocol, the eat-stop-eat protocol, and the warrior protocol. These four intermittent fasting protocols have been used and reused many times over a long time to effectively and efficiently attain their aims. These four protocols will be discussed in detail in this chapter.

A. The 16/8 Intermittent Fasting Protocol (The Lean Gains Method)

The 16/8 intermittent fasting protocol is a fasting protocol that involves putting a restriction on the number of foods consumed as well as beverages that are filled with calories for a total of 8 hours while getting off food completely for 16 hours every day. Although the more popular usage of the 16/8 protocol is done on a daily basis, the frequency can actually be set to daily, weekly, twice a week, or even just once. A major eyebrow-raiser in the 16/8 fasting method is the fact that one has to go a whole 16 hours without eating food. But this is not as harsh as it probably sounds. The 16 hours you have to abstain from food includes the time you spend sleeping (which in its own right could take up to 6 – 8 hours). If you subtract your sleeping time from the 16 hours of abstinence, then you may be left with a number that makes perfect sense to you and which you would be comfortable and willing to use.

The main foundations of the lean gains method are the fast, train hard in the fasted state, and then eat a large meal after the heavy training. This method of intermittent fasting became popular in recent times, particularly among people who want to shed some fat and lose weight. The lean gains method is unlike most other intermittent fasting protocols that are known to be tightly restrictive; it is much more flexible as it allows for more flexibility and is easier to follow. The 16/8 protocol can literally fit into any schedule and lifestyle and, therefore, does not require you to make any massive changes to your way of life. You only have to decide on the 8-hour' window' during which you would eat, and then fast for the remaining 16 hours. For example, you may choose to eat between 11:00 am and 7:00 pm and fast from 7:00 pm till 11:00 am the next day. Apart from the weight loss solution which the 16/8 method offers so effectively, it is also believed to have the capacity to help you achieve improved blood sugar levels, greater brain function, and long life.

The 16/8 intermittent fasting protocol caused quite a stir when it made its debut in the dietary world. While many people waved it aside and considered it another bit of diet fad, some others exaggerated its efficacy as a weight loss solution and blew it out of proportion. But soon thereafter, people started to realize the true potential of the lean gains method and how it can be applied to address various bodily issues. And as this happened, the number of people committing to the protocol grew exponentially.

In order to intermittent fast safely and healthily, you must endeavor to get and remain hydrated by drinking a lot of water while you are not in the eating window. If you are the coffee or tea type, then it is better and recommended that you take your coffee or tea in the morning, as it can give you the right level of energy to work out. Be sure not to add creamers to your coffee as it increases your calorie intake significantly. There is also a school of thought that states that ingesting a BCAA supplement just before your work out period can help you avoid muscle loss. When you get into the 8 hours eating window, it is of vital importance that you eat food that is of high quality and contain all of the necessary nutritional requirements (especially proteins, carbs, fat, minerals, and vitamins). You must guard against getting dehydrated throughout the fasting and eating periods and meet your daily protein requirements. This helps to prevent loss of muscle during the work out time. Take in as many proteins as you can during the eating window and take in carbs to provide those calories you would need to facilitate your work out. You may feel dizzy or weak if you don't fill up with enough calories.

While in the process of obtaining calories and getting ready to gain muscle, don't overeat just because you feel you are going to have to fast for 16 hours after the eating window closes. The purpose of intermittent fasting is to restrict your feeding and get your body in shape. If you deal in junk foods or binge-eat high-calorie foods that are devoid of essential nutrients, then you would be defeating the primary purpose of starting the intermittent fasting routine in the first place.

As with most diet control protocols, the 16/8 intermittent fasting protocol, though incredibly effective, has its own downsides. First, it might take some time for your body to be able to adjust to the new diet regimen, and so your body might respond in ways you don't expect. Secondly, if you are currently struggling with pathologies involving blood sugar level (such as diabetes or hypoglycemia), then this protocol of intermittent fasting may not be appropriate for you. Lastly, if you are a breastfeeding or pregnant woman, then you may need to discuss with your doctor on the suitability of the lean gains intermittent fasting protocol for you.

However, if you are not in any of the categories mentioned above, then you might as well kick0start your lean gains adventure already. Guidelines on the proper application of the lean gains intermittent fasting protocol will now be discussed further.

Guidelines for starting the 16/8 intermittent fasting protocol

The 16/8 intermittent fasting protocol should be applied according to the 8-hour eating and 16-hour fasting rule. During the 8-hour eating window, it is recommended that you at least eat two large meals or a large meal and two small meals, before which you should take about 10 grams of BCAA in order to optimize results. This is the general outline of the lean gains intermittent fasting protocol. However, as has been highlighted before now, the 16/8 fasting protocol is a flexible method and can, therefore, be tweaked to suit one's unique needs and circumstances. Here are sample setups of the 16/8 fasting protocol:

i.   **The typical 16/8 fasting protocol setup**

In this setup, the first meal of the eating window should be taken immediately after the workout and should be the largest meal of the day (the one with the most calories). The second meal may be taken a couple of hours after the first meal is ingested, and the last meal of the day before the fast may be consumed just before the end of the 8-hour fasting window. The overall setup for the protocol could be as thus:

- 11:30 am – 12 noon: Take about 10 grams of BCAA. You may also take it 5 to 15 minutes before your workout time.
- 12 noon – 1:00 pm: This is the workout window. Use this time to work out intensely.
- 1:00 pm: This is when you take your post-workout meal, the first and heaviest meal of the day.
- 4:00 pm: You should take your second meal of the day at this time. It could be another large meal or one of a two-part smaller meal.
- 9:00 pm: This is the eighth and final hour of the fasting window and the time to consume your last meal of the day before the fasting period.

Note that the total calories you have to consume during the course of the day should be spread throughout the day, as depicted in the example above.

ii.   The early morning training setup

One other notable thing that we can see from the above sample is that the start of the fasting window eats deep into the day, meaning that you would have to fast till almost noon if you were to implement the strategy. However, if you are an early riser and would rather exercise very early in the day (or if you are trying to get into that habit), then you may want to make certain modifications to the timings in the first example above. The sample setup below demonstrates these modifications:

- 6:00 am: Take about 10 grams of BCAA at this time. You could also take the supplement until about 5 – 15 minutes before your workout.
- 6:00 am – 7:00 am: This is your 1-hour workout window. Train intensely during this time.
- 8:00 am: Take another 10 grams of BCAA.
- 10:00 am: Take yet another 10 grams of BCAA.
- 12 noon – 1:00 pm: This is when you take your first post-workout meal, which is also the largest meal of the day. In addition, this marks the beginning of the feeding window.
- 8:00 pm – 9:00 pm: Take your last meal of the feeding window at this time. It is the last meal you'll take before the fasting period.

One thing is immediately striking from the example above: you only get to take two meals during the feeding period – a larger meal immediately after a workout and a smaller one just before the end of the feeding window and before the start of the fasting window. It is recommended that you consume the BCAA supplement in the form of powder instead of tablets. To do this, you could dissolve 40 grams of BCAA powder in a shake and divide the solution into three parts. Take one part of the solution in intervals of 2 hours starting from some 5 – 15 minutes before your workout. Although tabs are cheaper, taking tabs every time you want to work out could soon turn you into a pill popper, as you would need to take a lot of them in the course of your intermittent fasting journey.

iii.   The college student setup

The two sample setups detailed above are popular and are being utilized by many people who are interested in using the lean gains method. However, while they might be suitable for a great many people, some people don't take much liking to it. College students, for instance, or people who typically have a flexible working schedule would prefer to have a more flexible feeding regimen. Because the lean gains method is a particularly flexible fasting protocol, the people who fall in this category can tweak the protocol to suit their unique needs. The sample setup given below should suffice for people who want extra flexibility in their lean gains journey.

- 12 noon – 1:00 pm: This is when you must eat your first meal of the day (also called the pre-workout meal). Note that unlike the first meal in the earlier detailed sample setups, this is not your largest meal of the day. You may also take this meal around lunchtime. This meal should take about a quarter of your daily calorie requirement.
- 3:00 pm – 4:00 pm: Use this window to carry out your workout. If you elect to take your pre-workout meal at your usual lunchtime, then leave your workout till after a few hours after taking the meal.
- 4:00 pm – 5:00 pm: Take your post-workout meal at this time. This is your second and your largest meal of the feeding window.
- 8:00 pm – 9:00 pm: Take your last meal of the feeding window during this period.

This sample is similar to the first sample setup, where there are three meals taken during the fasting window, in which the total calorie requirements for the day are spread unevenly. One difference between this setup and the first lies in the absence of ingestion of BCAA supplement. The BCAA supplement is supposed to be administered to give your body nutrients to work on as your train. The pre-workout meal in this setup effectively nullifies the need for any further administration of BCAA.

iv.   Lean gains protocol setup for people with usual working hours

If you fall into the category of people who have normal working hours (you work from 9 am – 5 pm), then this setup should be suitable for you.

- 12 noon – 1:00 pm: Take your first meal of the day in this period. This is also your first pre-workout meal of the day. This meal should take up only as much as 25n percent of your daily calorie intake. You could also take this meal at your usual lunchtime.
- 4:00 pm – 5:00 pm: This is your second pre-workout meal and should be slotted into this period. This meal should take the same proportion of your daily calorie intake as the first meal.

- 8:00 pm – 9:00 pm: This is your post-workout and third meal. It is also your largest meal of the day, taking up as much as half of your daily calorie intake.

Benefits of the 16/8 intermittent fasting protocol

- **Reduced hunger levels:** This is perhaps one of the most important benefits of intermittent fasting in general to people who are looking to lose weight. One of the biggest roadblocks that people struggling with weight issues encounter is dealing with hunger. The feeling of hunger is a natural instinct that most people in the world have. When you skip breakfast – which is an underlying principle of the lean gains fasting protocol – your body responds by adapting to your new dietary pattern. The body's hormones, especially the hormone ghrelin, adapt to the new pattern so that you no longer feel the hunger in the morning. This adaptation occurs after about a week of your starting the protocol.
- **Meal planning becomes an easier routine:** With basically fewer meals to consume, you are left with fewer meals to plan and more time to spend on other activities.
- **Get lean faster:** The lean gains protocol is specifically designed to you to lose as much fat as you can while not changing your lifestyle massively. Fasted workout regimens and dietary protein supplements ensure that you get to your destination weight as soon as possible.

Who should and shouldn't use the 16/8 intermittent fasting protocol

It is a good thing to want to engage in intermittent fasting and an even better thing to have gone as far as choosing what protocol you would like to start on. However, you must know that the ultimate purpose of intermittent fasting is to bring about an improvement in our internal environment. Therefore, in order to ensure that you don't end up suffering more harm than reaping benefits from your intermittent fasting journey, you must ensure to adhere to certain health rules. As much as you may want to shred off that extra weight or gain muscle and get lean, quite unfortunately, the 16/8 fasting protocol may not be for you. Below are some of the circumstances under which you could proceed with your lean gains plans:

- **If you don't want to make wholesale changes to your dietary habit:** The dietary world has changed a lot in recent years. We have seen one diet fad after another spring up and take center stage in the media space. Most of these fad diets come with more restrictions and regulations than benefits and often require strict adherence to laid down rules. One of the beauties of the lean gains intermittent fasting protocol lies in its dietary flexibility – it doesn't attempt to dictate to you what you eat or what you can't. You simply have to restrict your feeding window and continue eating what you have always eaten. On the side of how much you are allowed to eat, as long as you are eating the number of calories your body can conveniently handle, there is really not much that the lean gains method has to say about that as well.

- **If you are a breakfast skipper, then the lean gains system is yours to try:** If you are like many people who would rather not consume any food on early mornings, then it might be easier to slip in the lean gains protocol into your diet schedule. Fasting from * PM till 12 noon the following, for instance, might already be a habit in your lifestyle; hence, practicing the setup might seem more or less like your routine lifestyle. What's more, if you like to take a sip or two of strong, black coffee before setting out to work, then you are in luck because the lean gains method permits the consumption of coffee, tea, and water during fasting periods. You could even add a teaspoon to your coffee cup if you see it fit to do so.

- **If you usually find yourself guilty of forgetting to eat lunch:** Sometimes you are so busy you forget to have lunch at the scheduled period. This 'offense' might become one too many if you work a job that takes up much of your afternoon. If you are this sort of person, then stop feeling guilty; the 16/8 protocol may be well suited to your lifestyle.

- **If you have issues making out time to cook and clean:** One of the most sought after benefits of the lean gains protocol is its flexibility and simplicity. No matter which lean gains setup you choose to start, you'll definitely be eating fewer meals than you used to. Fewer meals directly translate into fewer dishes you have to clean and a reduction in the time you spend cooking. With the lean gains protocol, you also don't have to spend time cooking complex new meals as you can literally stick to your existing meal plan during the feeding window.

- **If you are a community type of person:** It is a fact that the health habits of your friends can strongly influence your own. If you enjoy meeting and working with other people, then the lean gains protocol will be very well suited to you. You could start a community of fasting friends, join one, or simply ask if your best friend would like to go on the lean gains journey with you. This will go a long way in motivating you to stick to the plan.

- **If you have tried many other diets and haven't achieved your goal:** If you have tried out just about every diet out there and have not found the right one for you or are yet to reap the rewards you expect, then it might be time to try out the lean gains protocol. The lean gains protocol might work wonders where other diets have failed.

If you find that most of the points highlighted above do not in any way describe your kind of person or fit you, you might want to have a rethink about putting the lean gains protocol to the test. Even if the point above describes who you are, you still have to assess yourself further to find out if the lean gains if for you. You could assess yourself under the following points:

- **If you have certain medical conditions:** The lean gains method may not be suitable to you if you are struggling with certain health issues, such as nutritional deficiencies, menstrual problems, abnormally low weight, hypotension (low blood pressure), diabetes, and migraines. If you have any of these conditions, then for your own safety, make sure to consult your doctor before you think of starting on the lean gains.

- **If you have to drive or are in charge of handling heavy machinery:** Although people react differently to fasting, you may have symptoms of dizziness or lightheadedness during the fasting window, especially in the first few weeks after you start with the protocol. These effects are not ideal if you have to drive or operate heavy machinery. If you still want to proceed on the fasting protocol, then ensure that you stay off driving for the first week or two.

- **If you are planning to drink alcohol:** The absorption of alcohol is slowed by the presence of food in your stomach. According to the Mayo Clinic, your risk of alcohol poisoning is significantly increased when you drink on an empty stomach. Drinking alcohol immediately after fasting may put you at this risk. If you have a social event around the corner in which you are certain you'll be drinking alcohol, then it is best you let the event pass before you start your fasting regimen.
- **If you are taking certain medications:** If you are currently taking medications that you either have to take at the same time regularly or with a meal, then you might hold off on engaging in the lean gains. One such substance that is significantly affected by dietary changes is progestin-only birth control for contraception. The efficacy of this medication may be reduced if you make abrupt changes to your feeding habits. Some other medications that might be affected by fasting are blood thinners, anti-psychotics, transplant medications, and antidepressant drugs. Furthermore, it is vital for some drugs to be ingested with meals, such as fat-soluble vitamins (vitamins A, C, and E), certain drugs the absorption of which depends on food, and some drugs that may create an upset in the stomach. If you are on any medications, then be sure to consult your physician or pharmacist regarding how safe it is for you to begin the lean gains.
- **If you're trying to conceive:** Fasting may have a negative impact on fertility. Although there is a dearth of scientific evidence to support this hypothesis, if you are trying to get pregnant, perhaps it is better for you to stay off fasting at the moment. This recommendation holds true is you are pregnant or lactating as well.
- **If you just started taking a medication:** Certain drugs cause dizziness and lightheadedness, and fasting does not improve these symptoms. On the contrary, the side effects of fasting may exacerbate these symptoms. You should first allow your body to adapt to the new medication before you begin to pull it in the direction of intermittent fasting.
- **If you travel quite a lot:** Apart from the side effects of the lean gains protocol that affect any kind of lifestyle, lean gains is not suitable for certain lifestyles at all. You may find the lean gains protocol to be a wrong fit if you travel a lot. Incessantly changing your time zone and hanging out with colleagues for lunch in new locations are not perfect ingredients for adhering to a lean gains setup.
- **If your working schedule is not consistent:** The lean gains protocol needs to be applied on a consistent basis to produce optimum results. If you have an inconsistent working schedule that would not allow you to maintain a setup, then the lean gains may not yield optimum results for you.

Foods to eat and avoid on the 16/8 intermittent fasting protocol

The 16/8 protocol is not a dietary protocol that imposes any regulations on the sort of foods to eat. What is recommended is that you maintain a healthy diet that is rich in proteins and unprocessed foods. A lot of emphasis is placed on proteins in the lean gains protocol because proteins are filling and last longer in the body. Furthermore, the heating effect of food is also found to be greater with proteins than with other classes of food. Hence, digestion of protein results in a greater amount of fat burning. Additionally, your body requires protein to retain muscle tissue while burning fat.

Instead of focusing on the kinds of food to eat the lean gains protocol focuses on the times you consume food. As a general rule, it is recommended that you schedule your 16/8 set up in such way as to fast in the night hours and in the early hours of the day. Therefore, you may have to avoid late-night meals, midnight snacks, breakfast, and snacks in mid-morning. Also in the ideal setting, the 8-hour eating window should begin around noon and end at 8 PM. You may eat as many as 2 or 3 meals during this window.

The eating and fasting windows make sense the way they are scheduled; the 16-hour fasting window (stretching through the night and early morning) is a long enough period for the body to exhaust the glycogen deposit in the liver. Fasting for this long also serves to improve insulin sensitivity. On the flip side, the 8-hour fasting window is socially attractive. Many people like to eat lunch at work with friends and colleagues and eat dinner with family members. The feeding window ideally starts at noon and ends at 8 PM, a period during which these two important meals are likely to be consumed. The statement that breakfast is the most important meal of the deal is a myth that has been pushed by the media to promote cereals. Studies abound that show that skipping breakfast does not necessarily affect weight loss in any way.

Another area that the lean gain protocol focuses on is that of caloric intake. The lean gains protocol, though stressing the need to schedule feeding, does not recommend or suggest decreasing one's calorie consumption. You should eat sufficiently on training days and a bit less on rest days.

As for foods to avoid on the lean gains protocol, while the protocol does not expressly impose any food restrictions, it does express concerns over the consumption of smoothies, nuts, and dried fruits. Contrary to what many 'diet gurus' say about nuts and dried fruits, the lean gains protocol is not quick to support its consumption. It may be more beneficial to eat fish instead of nuts and dried fruits. Nuts contain greater caloric content than chocolate and are less filling. Dried fruits contain lots of sugar and fiber with little to no protein content. These substances create very little feeling of satiety and take a large chunk of our daily calorie intake. Thus, nuts and dried fruits, as well as smoothies, can be rightly described as a waste of calories. So, as convenient as they might seem, you may do better to avoid these and other foods that don't add much to your satisfaction and replace them with whole meals.

Tips for effectively applying the 16/8 intermittent fasting protocol

Here are key points to consider when using the lean gains intermittent fasting protocol. These tips should help get you on track and guide you through your lean gains adventure.

- You must ensure to not consume any calories during the fasting window of the protocol. This goes against the tenets of the protocol and may compromise your efforts and detract from your results. However, you may consume coffee, sweeteners that are devoid of calories, diet soda, and sugar-free gums (although they contain a number of calories, these substances are still considered OK). Putting a little bit of milk in your cup of coffee may not affect your results in any way as well (emphasis must be placed on "a little bit." A half or full teaspoon of milk per cup of coffee should be the maximum bit here). If you drink a lot of coffee in the course of a single day, then even this little measure of milk might eventually become too much and, therefore, detrimental. So, use milk toppings sensibly and appropriately. Sugar-free gum would also not affect anything, as long as you don't consume a massive chunk of it.

- Don't see the fasting period as a time to get clumsy, lazy, and idle. It is time to be active and productive. You need to get things done during the fasted phase. Don't sit around and wait until you the fasting window closes and you can eat food again. See the fasted state as an 'opportunity' phase; an opportunity to work out and develop your body and mind.

- The frequency of meals in the feeding window is largely irrelevant. It is true that many people prefer to take up to three meals during the feeding window. Our recommendation is that you take as many meals as is reasonable and comfortable for you.

- Make sure to ingest the majority of your daily calorie intake during the post-workout period. The post-workout period is the period after your intense daily workout. That means you should consume roughly 95% of your daily calorie intake after workout (for setups that include a totally fasted workout), about 80% of your daily calorie intake after workout (for setups that allow for one pre-workout meal), and 60% of your daily calorie intake after workout (for setups that consist of two pre-workout meals).

- Evaluate your circumstances before you choose a setup to utilize. Once you have started on a particular setup, ensure that you stick to it strictly; your feeding window must be constant, as should your fasting window. If you have started on a setup that allows you to break the fast at 11 am and beginning another fasting phase at 8 pm, then try as much as you can to keep up with the pattern every day. This is due to the ability of your body to respond to your diet patterns. When you keep a regular pattern, you make it easier for your body to get accustomed to the new dietary regimen.

- On days when you are resting, it is recommended that your first meal is your largest meal of the day. This comes in contrast to training days when your largest meal of the day should ideally be your post-workout meal. A good strategy that works is to make your first meal on rest days take up as much as 40% of your daily calorie intake. This meal must be highly rich in protein; it is not abnormal to consume as much as 100 grams of protein in this meal alone.

- If you don't fancy eating large meals as early as the time you take your first meal and would rather push it deep into the day (such as dinner with family), then, doing so does not pose any great harm. The trick here is to do what you feel comfortable with and are able to do on a consistent basis.

- The total amount of calories you consume ultimately depends on the purpose of undertaking the intermittent fasting protocol and the sort of day it is. Whether it's to lose fat, to gain muscle, or to achieve body re-composition will affect the number of calories you consume. In addition, carbs and total calorie intake should be higher while fat is lower on training days, and carbs and calorie intake should lower while fat is higher on rest days. However, protein intake should be high on all days, regardless of energy requirements.

- You should take these supplements daily to help you get better results: a good multivitamin, fish oil, vitamin D, calcium (the extra calcium can be bypassed if you consume dairy products daily).

- If you have elected to go on a fasted workout setup, then it is highly recommended that you take a BCAA supplement or an essential amino acid mixture. If you do not have the financial capacity to consume these supplements, however, or you simply do not feel like taking such 'complex' substances, then you can make do with some protein. The importance of taking protein before workout is that it increases your body's metabolism. This fact has been checked scientifically and found to be true. Studies have shown that taking proteins before working out can increase your resting energy expenditure (RER), due to the increase in muscle protein synthesis brought about by the consumption of pre-workout protein. In some studies, consuming pre-workout protein is more effective for muscle protein synthesis and beneficial to workout than ingesting carbs. This increased effect is brought about by the body's ability to move amino acids to exercising muscles, which may exacerbate protein synthesis for the next 48 hours. This effect is not attainable if you work out without dietary protein supplements, if you work out in a completely fasted state, or if you work out on carbs only. A hypothesis put forward by scientists is that dietary amino acids blunt the action of cortisol, an effect that is not found with carbs or total fasted states. This effect leads to a reduction in cortisol. A reduced level of cortisol means that protein synthesis is increased (since cortisol is known to inhibit the synthesis of protein while aiding its breakdown). In summary, you stand to gain a lot when you ingest a protein supplement prior to working out. Pre-workout protein leads to better protein synthesis and, due to its effect on metabolism, help burn fat faster. To optimize your results and achieve your fasting purpose quicker:
    - Take about 10 grams of branched-chain amino acids (BCAA) or essential amino acids (EAA) about 5 to 15 minutes prior to working out. This is the ideal method of taking pre-workout protein.
    - As an alternative to the above method, you could ingest 30 grams of whet protein as a substitute for BCAA or EAA. This amount of whet protein would yield about the same amount of BCAA as in the above option.
    - Break your fast immediately after a workout. This should be the start of your feeding window. It is vital that you break your fast at this time in order to consume your post-workout protein.
    - In an ideal situation, your post-workout meal should be your heaviest meal of the day. After taking this meal, you could then taper down your daily caloric intake throughout the rest of the day.
    - End your feeding window with a meal that is low in carbs and high in proteins. It is recommended that the protein you consume in this meal is a slow-digesting one, such as eggs or cottage cheese. You could also take meat with veggies high in fiber. Although meat digests quickly, the fiber content of the veggies would help to slow down digestion.

- Don't aim at choosing a protocol that many people find fascinating or effective. Instead, use a protocol that is best suited to your unique lifestyle and needs. For example, if you work from 9 to 5 at least five days a week and the only time you can train on weekdays is after working hours, then training in the fasted state may be inappropriate to your lifestyle. Instead, choose a protocol that allows for one or two pre-workout meals.
- Notice that each setup had its benefits and merits. You must be clear on your fasting goal before you set out to start on the 16/8 protocol.

Summary of the 16/8 intermittent fasting protocol

- All of the meals you have to consume on a day should be taken during an 8-hour window. Adhere to this window and do not go very much lower or higher than it.
- Many lean gains protocol setups are designed so that you skip breakfast and fast in the morning. This has been found to be more convenient and easier to adhere to.
- You are to avoid any good substance that has calories during the fasting window, except such substances as coffee, tea, and sugarless him.
- Your body might take as many as 4 – 7 days to get used to your new diet pattern. You will feel hunger pangs until your body finally adjusts to the new pattern. Be aware of this pothole and prepare against falling into it.
- Eat your largest meal immediately after a workout. It is advised that you don't stay for longer than 2 hours without eating after your workout.
- If you are to train in a fasted state, take 10 grams of BCAA 5 – 15 minutes prior to working out and take 10 grams of BCAA in intervals of 2 hours thereafter before your first meal.
- On training days, take the majority of your calories after the workout.
- Take more carbs and more calories on training days and fewer carbs and fewer calories on rest days.

Mistakes to avoid when using the 16/8 intermittent fasting protocol

You must ensure that you have a solid understanding of the 16/8 protocol for it is only through that that you can apply it effectively to achieve your desired results. Lack of understanding of the protocol may lead to the following mistakes:

- **Not consuming enough calories:** When you apply the lean gains protocol, you inadvertently subscribe to pushing your meal back into the day while skipping breakfast altogether. On the surface, this may seem as though you are forced to reduce your daily calorie, but it doesn't have to be so. You must endeavor to stick to your daily caloric intake by making up for the skipped breakfast in other meals. If you don't consume enough calories while engaged in intermittent fasting, your metabolism might get slowed down. In addition, to an inhibited metabolism, your body might not burn fat as much as you would like and you may end up losing some muscle (which defeats the purpose of the intermittent fasting).

- **Not being mindful of what you consume:** The lean gains protocol does not support dietary restrictions of whatever kind. In fact, one of the most renowned practitioners and developers of the lean gains protocol, Martin Berkhan, says that he consumes cheesecake, alcohol, and ice cream and sees no reasons not to. However, you must not get the impression that the lean gains method gives a free pass to indulge in dietary indiscipline. You can't healthily eat just about anything you can lay your hands on. That might be detrimental. You have to restrict your intake of simple carbohydrates and sugars during your feeding window and try to consume whole, unprocessed foods instead.

- **Not engaging in high-intensity workouts:** Cardio workouts have been praised as the ultimate fat burners. While this may be true, you must not rely completely on cardio workouts as the only means of shedding off fat. If you do too much cardio training, you may force your body to start to use your muscle tissue as protein to drive your cardio training. Instead of focusing on only one type of training, try to strike a balance with your cardio workouts by performing high-intensity strength workouts. When you balance your training this way, your body will optimize the fat burning process without resorting to metabolizing your muscle tissue.

- **Developing an obsession over your meals:** The early developers of the lean gains protocol designed it to prevent their diets from taking over their lives. You shouldn't allow yours to take over your life either. Don't stress too much over maintaining a diet. If you must take a bar of chocolate outside of your feeding window, then just take it. It wouldn't change much. You could simply get back on track the next day. Stressing too much over getting slightly off track can lead you to feel guilty, further defaulting and ultimately giving up on your new adventure. Don't let this be your story. If there is a social function that you must attend and eat in, go right ahead and do just that. The aim of the lean gains protocol is to make your life simpler not harder or more stressful. The trick is to keep the number of times you fall off track few and far between and to get back on track as soon as you veer off it.

B. The 5:2 Intermittent Fasting Protocol

The 5:2 intermittent fasting protocol (also known as 'the fast diet' and would be referred to as such henceforth) is presently one of the most popular protocols of intermittent fasting in the dietary world. It is widely believed to have been initially developed and popularized by a British journalist and physician who goes by the name Michael Mosley. The fast diet protocol garnered public interest after Mosley made public his research on the health benefits of fasting on a BBC documentary program. Public interest in the fast diet went viral after he published a series of books on the protocol, the first of which is *the 5:2 Fast Diet*, published in early 2013.

The typical setup of the fast diet is such that you are allowed to eat as you normally would for 5 days in the week and 'fast' for two non-consecutive days. The fasting days are not total fasting days, as the protocol allows you to eat as much as 500 calories worth of food during the course of the day. Hence, a more befitting term for the fasting days would be calorie-restricted days, as the dieter is required to downsize the sheer amount of food they consume. Much like the lean gains fasting protocol, the fast diet is very flexible in terms of the kinds of food to eat. Restrictions are not placed on the sort of food to eat but the times in which food should be eaten. This makes the fast diet more of a lifestyle than a diet. This flexibility makes the fast diet more attractive to people venturing into intermittent fasting than most other diets.

Unlike on total fasting days, the calorie-restricted days in the fast diet involve eating a portion of the dieter's normal total caloric intake. The typical caloric intake on fasting days for a dieter on the fast diet is about a quarter of 25 percent of the normal daily calorie intake. For example, if your normal total caloric intake is 2,000 calories, then you would be required to eat only 500 calories on fasting days while on the fast diet. Therefore, you would be taking your usual 2,000 calories on normal days and 500 calories on each of your fasting days.

Another point to note is the setup of the fasting days. It is highly recommended by nutritionist and health experts that the fasting are kept apart and not consecutive. This is to make sure that the body is not starved for too long of its vital nutritional requirements. A typical setup is to keep the fasting days about 3 to 4 days apart; that is, for example, fasting on Monday and Thursday or Tuesday and Friday. This in itself further stretches the flexibility of the fast diet and, therefore, increases its appeal. This is one of the reasons the fast diet has been so popular among people who are jumping onto the intermittent fasting bandwagon. One other area of flexibility in the fast diet is the frequency of meals. No restrictions are placed on the number of meals you can eat on fasting and normal days or how frequently you can eat these meals. That is basically up to you to decide. You can decide how frequently you want to eat or eat as many times as you deem fit as long as you stick to the 25 percent rule on fasting days.

One major difference between the fast diet and lean gains protocol is while the lean gains restricts calorie intake for 16 hours of the day every day, the fast diet restricts calorie intake throughout a single day after which the dieter is allowed to go back to their normal feeding routine for the next day or few days before embarking on another day of calorie restriction. Because of the increased spacing between the bouts of calorie restriction, people on the fast diet should feel less severe pangs of hunger and have it easier to maintain their diet.

It may be tempting to overeat on normal days either as a sort of reward for cutting calorie consumption or as preparation for the calorie-restricted days. You must not do this. You should endeavor to maintain a healthy feeding lifestyle on normal eating days. Although no restriction is placed on the sort of food you can consume on the fast diet; it is generally recommended that you ingest lots of leafy green vegetables, lean meat, soups, eggs, coffee (particularly black coffee), tea, and water.

Benefits of the 5:2 Intermittent Fasting Protocol

The primary aim of the fast diet is to help you attain and maintain a healthy lifestyle and improve your general state of wellness. The fast diet is primarily based on the assumption that relatively short periods of fasting have a capacity to nudge the body into repairing damages while not entering into a starvation mode of energy conservation. Although this theory has not been proved beyond reasonable doubts, some clinical studies have been done to support the health benefits of the protocol. More research is needed on this subject matter to conclusively prove the much-asserted benefits of the fast diet. Some of the areas where the fast diet has shown promise are as follows:

- **The fast diet improves insulin sensitivity and kicks against type 2 diabetes:** For people with a body mass index over 25, the fact that the fast diet increases insulin sensitivity is a matter of vital importance and makes this protocol of the most appropriate intermittent fasting protocols for them. This benefit also works well for people suffering from borderline diabetes (prediabetes) or diabetic people who are not cyrrentl6 taking medications to reduce their blood sugar level. The fast diet is good to these groups of people, especially those who prefer to deal with single days of extreme calorie reduction to slight reductions in calorie intake on a daily basis.

  The effect of the 5:2 fasting protocol on type 2 diabetes is not just another high assumption; it has been backed by scientific studies. One Australian study published in July 2012 sought answers to the question of whether the fast diet was indeed beneficial to those suffering from type 2 diabetes. The authors, from the University of South Australia, conducted a trial that lasted about 12 months (a very long time for a weight loss study) on 137 individuals suffering from type 2 diabetes. Coupled with their diabetic condition, these individuals were also overweight. The study was aimed at comparing the effects of a 5:2 diet with those of a typical calorie-restricting diet on weight loss. The research subjects were separated into two groups. Both groups were offered meal menus from which they chose and ate real food and guided by a dietician at the start of the study. Overall, it was a very pragmatic approach.

  The researchers collected the weight data of the study participants and found out that the group on the 5:2 diet had on average lost about 15 pounds of weight while the control group had lost about 11 pounds on average. Other factors, such as motivation, were also taken into consideration. For instance, more the determined individuals were found to have lost more weight than the less determined ones. In addition, the group on the fast diet were also observed to have lost about 40 percent more body fat than their control counterparts. Among the test group, some individuals showed improvements in blood sugar control and were able to reduce their medication.

- **The fast diet may help prolong the onset of dementia:** Although there is an obvious dearth of research about the effects of intermittent fasting on the brains of humans, there have been bold attempts at unraveling the effects of fasting on animal brains. One such researcher who has delved into the effects of diet fasting on the brain health of animals is Dr. Mark Mattson of the National Institute on Ageing situated in Baltimore.

  Dr. Mattson had in his laboratory mice that had undergone genetic engineering, which rendered them vulnerable to dementia. In fact, at a year old (which is equivalent to the middle age in humans), these mice started to show signs of dementia by failing to solve simple problems when put in a maze. However, the scientist treated some of the mice in his lab to intermittent fasting. He discovered that these mice did not show any signs of dementia even after two years. Indeed, the earliest detectable signs of dementia in the mice on intermittent fasting began to appear towards their lives. If this is translated into human terms, it means that the humans would have started to show signs of dementia at the age of 90 – rather than the average 50.

These results, although obtained in animals much smaller and much less complex than we are, are signs that the fast diet can be effective in tackling the dementia problem. At the time of this writing, Dr. Mattson is currently attempting to try out his experiment on humans and might be publishing the result of that study soon.

- **The fast diet could reduce the risk of cancer:** In 2013, two researchers, Dr. Michelle Harvie working at the Genesis Breast Cancer Prevention Centre and Professor Tony Howell, conducted a scientific study on the efficacy of intermittent fasting in reducing the risk of cancer. The study consisted of a total of 115 women who were overweight and had a family history of breast cancer. The research subjects were divided into three groups.

  One of the study groups were treated to a low-calorie diet which consisted of fruits, vegetables, nuts, and fish. The diet plan also included olive oil, meat, and dairy. The second group of subjects was placed on the fast diet, where they are in their usual manners for 5 days in a week and had reduced calorie intake on the other two days. This group stuck to healthy meals on the normal days and a low carbohydrate 650-calorie meal on each of the calorie-restricted days. The last group was not placed on any comprehensive diet plans, except that they were instructed to avoid carbs for two days in a week.

  After three months had passed, the researchers collected weight data on the subjects. The results of the data collected showed that the subjects of the fast diet which restricted their calorie intake for 2 days a week recorded massive weight losses. On average these subjects lost about 11 pounds with some losing as much as over 40 pounds, in contrast to the average weight loss in subjects that were treated to standard diets, which stood at 8 pounds. Furthermore, the subjects on the fast diet lost twice as much body fat as the subjects on a standard diet lost. They also recorded massive drops in insulin levels – they had about 40 percent reduction in insulin levels compared to the other groups.

  The massive reduction in the levels of insulin recorded in subjects that were treated to the fast diet is important in the cancer prevention game because higher insulin levels increase cancer risk, especially breast cancer. High insulin levels also increase the risk of type 2 diabetes.

The benefits stated above are some of the positives of the fast diet. In addition to the above mentioned specific benefits you stand to gain from the fast diet, you also accrue regular intermittent fasting benefits, including weight loss, fat burning, dietary discipline, and overall body health improvement. The following points are more pros of the fast diet and should give you the gentle nudge you are waiting for onto the plains of the fast diet.

- **You don't ever have to go a full day without eating:** As earlier stated, the fast diet is so set up that it does not require you (nor does it recommend) to go on 24-hour total fasting. If you are in the working class and have concerns about how you are going to cope with fasting, then you need not worry. You could schedule the 2 days you have to restrict your calorie intake to one of the weekdays and one day in the weekend – Wednesday and Saturday, for example. This makes perfect sense. Of course, the diet is flexible, so you can tweak the setup as you see fit. All you should know is that you never have to go for a whole day without eating at all.

- **You are in total control of the setup:** This is becoming a repetition, but it's worth reiterating because it adds do much attractiveness to the fast diet. You can design your setup as you wish to suit your unique circumstances. You can choose which days to go on calorie restriction and which days to do your normal meals. It's all up to you. However, it is wise to not fast on consecutive days. Fasting back to back has its benefits, but it could get you burnt out quickly or lead you to binge after the days of restriction. It might also be detrimental if you are on a physically-demanding job. A simple rule of thumb is to spread the restriction days apart. How far apart depends entirely on you.
- **You can enjoy your favorite meals without feeling guilty:** With the fast diet, you can eat whatever it is you have been eating. You don't need to stop consuming your favorite meals and don't have to learn to prepare complex 'healthy' meals. The fast diet is as flexible as it gets. Remember, though, that you still have to keep a healthy diet.

The pros of the fast diet could take up an entire book of its own because they are numerous and seemingly unending. However, as with all intermittent fasting protocols, the fast diet has its own cons. Some of these cons are stated as follows:

- **There is no full fasting in the fast diet:** As much as it could be an advantage for some people, not attaining a full fast may be a disadvantage to certain people, especially those who are looking to lose weight rapidly. If you are suffering from high blood sugar, then the calorie restriction on fasting days may not cut it for you as you still have to eat well on those days. Hence, the blood sugar level could still rise on these days. This may not be congruent with your plan.
- **You may experience pangs of hunger:** Although you don't fast completely on fasting days, you may still find yourself feeling severely hungry as your body may not be acclimated to consuming such small calories. Some people have even reported that reducing their calorie intake makes them feel more hunger than fasting completely. This may be true because, with total fasting, your body finds a way to adjust to a lack of food if you keep fasting for a number of days or weeks. With the fasting diet, because you still eat on the fasting days, the time it takes your body to make this adjustment might be longer.

Sample Diet Plan to try on the 5:2 Intermittent Fasting Protocol

The fast diet protocol is one that can be correctly stated as a '5 days off, 2 days on' protocol. You are permitted to eat your normal daily calorie intake for 5 of the 7 days in a week while taking 25% of your daily calories on the remaining 2 days. But exactly how much calories is 'normal'? According to experts, the normal daily calorie intake for an adult male is 2400 calories and 2000 calories for an adult female. That means you would consume 2400 calories (2000, if you're a female) on each of the normal days and 600 calories (500, if you're a female) on each of the fast days. Here, we are going to look at a complete sample meal plan for all 7 days of a week on the fast diet.

While you may or may not stick to the plan given here, the aim of this plan is to help guide you through the journey, not to be a prescription. The plan aims to give a rounded approach to the fast diet protocol; the meals contained herein are designed to offer all of your body's nutritional requirements while making sure not to compromise your weight loss purpose. If after trying out the meal plan, you realize that you are not losing as much weight as you would like, then try to tweak things a little bit and see what happens. A common recommendation is to maintain your calorie intake on fast days but reduce that of your normal days.

You may reduce your normal-day calorie intake to 1600 (for females) or 2000 (for males), for example, and see where that takes you. Further reducing your fast day calorie intake might prove detrimental to your health. This diet plan does not specify the days of the week to eat normally or fast; it is recommended that you pick your own days. Furthermore, depending on how close your diet plan gets to your daily calorie limit, you could have some calories to spare on drinks, snacks, and some extra foods. The following is a meal plan for an entire week:

In this plan, we are going to schedule the calorie restriction days for the third and sixth days of the week. First, let's take a look at a meal plan for the 5 'normal' days, and afterward, delve into sample diet plans for the two fast days.

a. The 5 normal days

Day 1: 1630 calories

Breakfast: Delicious cream cheese plus raspberries

Get a toast of 2 slices of bread and spice it up with 30 grams of cream cheese plus 20 raspberries.

Lunch: Smoked Salmon with Egg Salad and Avocado

Half 3 cherry tomatoes and top with 75 grams of mixed leaf salad. Add a quarter sliced red onion, half avocado, a hard-boiled egg and 3 slices of smoked salmon. If you wish, you may sprinkle about 25 grams of walnuts on the salad, or keep them as snacks for later in the day.

Dinner: Chicken Fajitas with Potato Wedges

Take 120 grams of frozen potato wedges and cook in the oven according to packet instructions). Make your Chicken Fajitas and serve with the potato wedges. You should make two servings of Chicken Fajitas. Take one now and tuck the other in the refrigerator for a quick lunch tomorrow. Leftovers are a great way of saving time and energy on the fast diet and make the diet simpler.

Day 2: 1578 calories

Breakfast: Mushroom and tomato omelet plus baked beans

Mix 2 medium eggs and 1 tablespoon semi-skimmed milk with one pinch of pepper. Take a tablespoon of oil and fry four, button mushrooms in it for about 1 minute. Then, pour the eggs into the fryer. When you notice that the eggs are beginning to set, put in 3 cherry tomatoes (which you would have halved beforehand). Season as per your wish and get under the grill to finish up. Serve meal with half a can of baked beans.

Lunch: Leftover chicken fajita from day 1

Leftovers are a vital part of this diet plan because they save time and make the entire plan simpler. You could either warm up the leftover chicken fajita from day 1 or eat it cold. You may also enjoy the meal with a little dessert, such as bananas, or save the dessert and eat it as a snack later in the day.

Dinner: Quick Bolognese plus penne and parmesan

First, you should make the sauce for the quick Bolognese. Enjoy your Bolognese with 75 grams of dry weight penne and 1 tablespoon of parmesan. You could make 2 servings of this; eat one today and keep the other for the first fast day (the next day). A way to do this while being wary of calorie count is to divide the entire Bolognese meal into three parts. Eat two parts today and keep the third part in the fridge.

Day 3 (first fast day): We have planned out 12 meal ideas for the fasting days. These will be given in detail in the next section.

Day 4: 1615 calories

Breakfast: Grilled BLT sandwich

Put about 2 rashers of lean back bacon to grill. Then, prepare a sandwich using 2 slices of wholemeal bread, 2 leaves of lettuce, bacon, 1 tomato, and 1 teaspoon of mayonnaise.

Lunch: Greek salad

Prepare a Greek salad using any recipe of your choice, but make sure to use one that keeps the calorie count in check. You can include a banana for dessert or save it and eat it as a snack later.

Dinner: Sausage & mash plus onion gravy with veggies

Put about 200 grams of potato on fire and boil it until soft, then mash it. At about the same time, fry in 1 tablespoon of oil 3 pork sausages together with a whole sliced onion. Prepare 2 tablespoons of gravy granules using the instructions on the pack and add it to the frypan while stirring continuously to thicken. Serve this with the potato mash together with a bag of any steam veggies of your choosing.

Day 5: 1611 calories

Breakfast: Toasted bagel plus cheese

Toast 1 wholemeal bagel sliced in half. On getting toasted, spread 30 grams of cream cheese on it and enjoy the meal with 1 apple. If you would rather have it as a snack, then you may save the apple for later.

Lunch: Jacket potato plus beans and cheese

Bake about 200 grams of potato and top it with half a can of baked beans and about 30 grams of cheese. Serve the meal with a side salad constituted of 80 grams of mixed salad leaves and a quarter of chopped cucumber, plus a teaspoon of balsamic.

Dinner: Rice and chicken jalfrezi plus poppadoms with mango chutney

Use a suitable recipe to prepare the rice and chicken jalfrezi. But make sure that you keep the calorie constituent in check, especially if you'd be adding any more ingredients than what is considered typical. Make two servings of this meal. Eat one now and keep the other in the refrigerator for future use.

Day 6 (second fast day): We have planned out 12 meal ideas for the fasting days. These will be given in detail in the next section.

Day 7: 1607 calories

Breakfast: Tomato and spinach omelet

Mix together 1 teaspoon of milk and 2 medium eggs together and add a little amount of pepper. Heat some oil in the frying pan and then pour the egg mixture into the fryer. Once you realize the eggs are about to set, half 3 cherry tomatoes and get them into the mix. Then add about 60 grams of spinach and cook until you see that the spinach has wilted. Serve with half a can of baked beans.

Lunch: Leftover rice and chicken jalfrezi

This is the time to eat that rice and chicken jalfrezi you have been storing up since day 5. Simply heat it up and have a go at it. Easy!

Dinner: Breaded lemon sole plus petit pois and chips

Prepare a breaded lemon sole and about 150 grams of frozen chips in an oven (according to the instructions on the packet). Serve with about 80 grams of petit pois.

    b. Sample meal plans for the 2 fast days

Here are 12 sample meal plan ideas for the fast days of the 5:2 protocol:

Meal #1: 497 calories

Breakfast: whole meal toast plus peanut butter

Prepare a toast of a slice of wholemeal bread and take with a spread of 1 tablespoon of peanut butter.

Lunch: Some leftover quick Bolognese from day 2

Now you can get that quick Bolognese out of the fridge, warm up, and have it for lunch.

Dinner: Chicken noodle soup

Boil about 400ml of water and dissolve a cube of chicken stock in it to make a broth. Slice half a stalk of celery and half a carrot. Fry for a short time with 50 grams of roasted chicken breast. Get it the stock, put in 10 grams of egg noodles, and then bring the mix to a boil. Then, simmer for about 15 to 20 minutes.

Meal #2: 503 calories

Breakfast: Porridge plus blueberries

Prepare the porridge using 30 grams of oats, 100ml of water, and 75ml of semi-skimmed milk. Top the mix and serve with 45 to 50 blueberries.

Lunch: Vegetable soup

Put about 300 grams of fresh vegetable soup to heat and serve.

Dinner: Baked cod plus broccoli

Before getting anything into it, heat the oven to a temperature of 180 degrees Celsius. Take 80 grams of broccoli and chop it into florets and put the chops together with 140 grams of cod fillet into a baking dish. Crush half garlic on the cod fillet, and then drizzle with one tablespoon of oil. Season to taste. Bake the mix for about 8 – 10 minutes, then pop it under the grill for another 3 minutes. Serve the meal with some fresh lime juice.

Meal #3: 525 calories

Breakfast: Forty grams of Quaker Oats porridge

Prepare the porridge as per the instructions on the pack.

Lunch/Dinner: Beetroot and feta salad

Prepare the meal using 50 grams of beetroot, 30 grams of feta, 60 grams of spinach, and a squeeze of lemon juice. You may add an apple and a tablespoon of almond butter to the meal.

Meal #4: 430 calories

Breakfast: Sweet plums and yogurt

Prepare a meal of sweet plum and yogurt. You can tailor the recipe to your needs and wants, but use not more than 100 grams of low-fat yogurt, 2 plums, and a tablespoon of honey.

Lunch/Dinner: Ryvita and tuna slices

Use 2 Ryvita crackerbreads, 60 grams of tuna mayo, cracked black pepper, and sprinkle 70 grams of arugula on the mix. Take miso soup as a snack.

Meal #5: 478 calories

Breakfast: Soft boiled egg plus asparagus

Treat yourself to a meal of asparagus with soft boiled egg using 1 egg and 5 asparagus pieces. Season with salt and pepper to taste.

Lunch/Dinner: Turkey burgers and corn-on-the-cob

This makes for quite an interesting meal. Beat about 110 grams of turkey mince with one small egg, an onion, garlic, and chili. Serve with one corn-on-the-cob. Take a few frozen grapes as a snack.

Meal #6: 493 calories

Breakfast: Belvita breakfast biscuits packet (muesli)

Lunch/Dinner: Roasted veggies and balsamic glaze

Prepare the delicacy with half courgette, half aubergine, half butternut squash, and half red pepper. Add a tablespoon of balsamic vinegar and pour in a squeeze of lemon juice. Have Harley's sugarless jelly pot as a snack.

Meal #7: 419 calories

Breakfast: Spinach omelet

Prepare spinach omelet with 2 eggs and 60 grams of spinach leaves. Season with salt and pepper to taste.

Lunch/Dinner: Hummus and crudites

Make the meal with 40 grams of hummus, a small to medium bowl of carrots, cucumber, and pepper. Take 60 grams of Edamame beans and rock salt as a snack.

Meal #8: 452 calories

Breakfast: low-fat yogurt with banana

The meal should contain about 100 grams of low-fat yogurt and a banana. Sprinkle cinnamon on top and serve.

Lunch/Dinner: Turkey breasts and wilted spinach

Prepare the meal with 125 grams of turkey breast steak and a cup of cooked and salted spinach. Have 10 grams of popcorn as a snack.

Meal #9: 422 calories

Breakfast: Smoothie of apple, ginger, and carrot

Prepare a smoothie from 1 apple, 1 carrot, and raw ginger.

Lunch/Dinner: Pitta pizza

Prepare the meal from Weight Watchers wholemeal pitta, 25 grams of Extra Light Philadelphia cheese, 1 tomato, and mixed herbs. Season with salt and pepper to taste. Have 100 grams of blueberries and a fistful of almonds as a snack.

Meal #10: 489 calories

Breakfast: Mixed berry bowl

Prepare the bowl with about 100 grams of strawberries, 100 grams of raspberries, and 100 grams of blueberries.

Lunch/Dinner: Harissa chicken plus chargrilled veggie couscous

Prepare the meal from 1 chicken breast (weighing about 130 grams), 100 grams of veggie couscous, and a tablespoon of harissa paste. Take 10 pistachios as a snack.

Meal #11: 424 calories

Breakfast: Take 3 pancakes (the *Weight Watchers Blueberry Buttermilk Pancakes* is highly recommended) for breakfast.

Lunch/Dinner: Roasted red pepper and tomato soup plus Ryvita crackerbreads

Prepare the meal from 2 original Ryvita crackerbreads, half tomato, half onion, half red pepper, garlic, 1 tablespoon of tomato puree, half a tablespoon of cumin, Oxo chicken, stock cube, salt, and half a tablespoon of balsamic vinegar. Season with pepper to taste. Have a tablespoon of pumpkin and sunflower seeds as a snack.

Meal #12: 506 calories

Breakfast: Fruit and nut muesli

Lunch/Dinner: Pesto salmon plus curly kale

Prepare the meal from 100 grams of salmon fillet, 3 tablespoons of green pesto, and about 100 grams of the combination of steamed kale and black pepper. Have 60 grams of stoned cherries as a snack.

Tips for Kick-Starting and maintaining the 5:2 Intermittent Fasting protocol

No matter how flexible and achievable the fast diet may seem, you may still find that it is harder to sustain than your normal lifestyle. Many people venturing into the fast diets see themselves quitting after sometime largely because they did not anticipate or get adequate knowledge of what to expect in the course of the regimen. Starting on the fast diet only to quit it and revert to your routine lifestyle may harm your readiness and willingness to try out any such dietary regimens in the future. Hence, the issues you have to solve with intermittent fasting remains and may even deteriorate. Here are some tips that are sure to help you get the most out of your fast diet regimen.

- **Keep yourself busy:** You are more likely to feel pangs of hunger when you are inactive and bored than when you are actively engaged in an activity. Keep yourself away from the temptation of ruining your fast by getting busy. Go for a walk, read a book, or visit a friend. Do something that takes your mind away from the hunger.
- **Maintain a hydrated state:** Water barely contains any calories, yet it can make you feel full for a long stretch of time. Water can also help prevent headaches – which are common side effects of partial and total fasting. Get into the habit of drinking water before and after meals as it makes you feel fuller than when you don't. You could also make a cup of black coffee or tea on your fasting days when you are feeling hungry. These can get you filled up and keep you on track. If you'll be adding some milk in your drinks, then take note of the number of calories you consume from it, and account for it as part of your daily allowed calorie intake.
- **On fasting days, eat only when you're really hungry:** If you are used to getting hold of a chocolate bar at the slightest rumbling of your stomach, you might need to hold off on that habit for now. You don't want to waste calories on foods that don't really fill you up when you have such an extreme calorie restriction to stick to. The fast diet is primarily about training your body to strive without much food. Just by eating lunch 2 hours after the usual time can help your body adapt to fasting for a long time.
- **On normal days, don't eat too much:** Although you may be tempted to view your normal days as an opportunity to consume as much as you wish, your body could become confused if you eat more than is necessary – on one day you're training your body to hold hunger for long periods of time and on another day you're treating your gut to a feast. This may prolong your body's adaptation period.
- **Know yourself:** The internet is rife with information about how to go about maintaining a healthy dietary lifestyle. Some nutritionists may tell you that it is best to consume three square meals every day while others may tell you to skip breakfast. The trick to avoiding confusion is to know your body and what works for you. If you're already used to skipping

breakfast, then your body would have adjusted such that it doesn't expect any food early in the morning. What's more, skipping breakfast allows you to save calories and have more substantial meals for lunch and dinner.

- **Veggies and protein are your best bet:** Eat mostly veggies and protein on your fasting days as they make you feel fuller for longer while making sure you don't lack basic nutrients.
- **Plan for your fasting days:** Make adequate plans for what to eat on your fasting days. This way, you'll avoid having to grab any nearby chocolate bars when you are hungry.
- **Get junk-proof:** Always have a healthier substitute for junk food around and at reach. As much as you may want to keep a healthy lifestyle and eat only carefully prepared meals on fasting days, you may find that you simply don't have the time to prepare meals sometimes. If you have healthy snacks around in these times, they may save you from falling into the junk trap.
- **Good schedules are key:** It is wise to schedule your fasting days for when you'll be busy but not feasting or having friends over. Use this schedule for a week or two and see if it would suit you moving forward or you if you'll need to create another one.
- **Get disciplined:** This is perhaps the most important tip of all. As long as you are in possession of a stomach, the hunger pangs will come, there's nothing to do about that. But they will go soon after. You need to understand this and prepare to face it.
- **Don't play the guilt game:** Consuming 515 calories instead of the recommended 500 wouldn't cause any great change. Don't feel guilty for not adhering strictly to the calorie restriction. The aim is to stay around the recommended calories, and as long as you can achieve that, you're right on track.
- **Be clear on your 'why':** Before you set out to fast – and to be able to gain maximum efficacy from your fasting regimen – you need to be clear on why you want to do it in the first place. If you are in it because it is currently trending or because someone you know or respect is trying it out, then there is the danger of it turning into yet another fad diet for you. Whether it is to lose some of the weight you're carrying, assisting you to improve your insulin resistance or to reduce your risk of Alzheimer's disease, you must know exactly why you are in the fasting game otherwise you may not have enough motivation and willpower to see it through.
- **Make the best choice of meals:** On your fast days, be sure to consume foods that are nutritious and filling but low in calories. You could literally eat a ton of these and not exceed your calorie restriction. Some of the best foods to eat on fasting days are non-starchy veggies, (avoid potatoes, peas, and corn), lean proteins including eggs and chicken, berries, and plain (Greek) yogurt.
- **Spice things up a bit:** While it may be simpler and easier to stick to one meal plan and basically eat the same set of foods on fast days, it may get a little boring and bland to keep consuming the same foods after some time. You should be creative with meals. Get different menus and try them out one after the other. Chances are, after trying out various meals, you will get yourself some favorites that you can stick with throughout your fasting journey. You can ensure that you never exceed your calorie limit by a lot by using calorie-

tracking software available all over the internet. Some of this software even allows you to build your own unique recipes.

C. The Eat-Stop-Eat Protocol

The eat-stop-eat protocol is a nice way to go if you are trying out intermittent fasting for the first time. Many people who have tried one intermittent fasting or another find the idea of having to restrict food intake or put a stop to eat completely for a set period of time daunting and highly inconvenient. This is one of the leading reasons why some people quit an intermittent fasting protocol shortly after starting on it. The eat-stop-eat protocol is designed to address this problem by making intermittent fasting more comfortable and less stressful. This protocol is a modified version of the alternate day fasting, which was brought to life by the fitness and nutrition expert Brad Pilon. In brief, the eat-stop-eat protocol requires that you fast for a period of 24 hours once or twice a week.

What has become the eat-stop-eat protocol is an idea that grew out the graduate thesis of its founder, Brad Pilon at the University of Guelph, Ontario, Canada. Although he initially stated that he does not have any intentions of defending the benefits of intermittent fasting, Pilon's efforts at developing the eat-stop-eat protocol ended up doing just that. It was noted early on by Pilon that most of the intermittent fasting protocols were too focused on the fasting part while paying little to no attention to the feasting part. According to him, this overemphasis placed on fasting may as well result in as much stress as can be created by routine calorie-restricting diets. This does not help those on a diet. The eat-stop-eat diet was created to make fasting as flexible as possible for everyone and rid it of stress.

The primary tenet of the diet, as is the case with most other intermittent fasting protocols, is the shift of emphasis from what to eat and what not to eat to when to eat. This shift in focus is done with an aim to reduce the stress caused by regular weight-loss diets. As mentioned earlier, the protocol requires that you fast for a whole day. However, this fasting day only comes once or twice in a week or two, thereby creating flexibility. On fasting days of the diet, you can take drinks that don't contain any calories, and on normal days you can eat pretty much anything you want. goes. The ideal result of the protocol is to make you lose body fat while retaining muscle mass, and all this without having to think about food too much. In addition, you stand to gain tons of other benefits that the protocol has been scientifically proven to offer. These benefits include, but are not limited to, cell renewal and cleansing, reduced risk for diabetes, reduced risk for cardiovascular diseases, and reduced risk for Alzheimer's disease.

How to start on the Eat-Stop-Eat protocol

Almost anyone can start on the eat-stop-eat protocol – that's how simple and convenient it is. However, this protocol may be better suited to dieters who are in need of a more flexible dietary protocol. It is also a good fit for dieters who are not likely or willing to let go of their favorite meals. The eat-stop-eat protocol gives you more freedom as you start or continue on your quest to shed body fat.

The major requirement of this protocol is that you fast for a period of 24 hours once or twice a week. When you schedule, these fasting days are entirely dependent upon your personal preferences. It is generally recommended that the fasting days (if two) are non-consecutive days of the week. Its flexibility also means that you can start fasting any time you feel is convenient for you. For instance, if you can't do without having breakfast, then you can have breakfast as 6:30AM on a fasting day. Then you fast from that time till 6:30AM the next day. This counts as a whole day fast.

On a similar note, if you feel strongly about dinner, then you can dine with your family at 8PM on a fast day. That means you would have to eat at 8PM the following day. It's really that convenient. You could even fix your fasting days as per your social commitments. For example, if you were planning to start your fasting day at 7AM today and a client called and requested that you grab lunch with them, you can attend that lunch meeting with no worries if you are on the eat-stop-eat protocol. All you have to do is reposition your start time to sometime after that lunch. The eat-stop-eat protocol can effectively be defined around two words: flexibility and convenience. If these words are what you are looking for in a dietary regimen, then you have arrived at the right protocol.

The eat-stop-eat protocol is similar to the alternate day fasting, only more flexible and more convenient. It doesn't come with a list of dos and don'ts. All you have to do is schedule 2 fasting days in a week. Eat whatever you normally eat on non-fasting days and abstain from eating or drinking anything that contains calories on the fasting days. And you must stick to this schedule. As much as this protocol is easy to start and adhere to, it comes with a few challenges of its own.

One of the challenges you are likely to face on this diet is hunger pangs that will arise as a result of fasting. However, because, unlike some other intermittent fasting protocols where fasting is done daily, fasting is not done on a daily basis in the eat-stop-eat protocol. This might make your body take longer to adjust to your new dietary pattern. While your body is trying to adjust, side effects such as headaches and irritability may set in and make your fasting more hectic than it should ideally be. Another challenge you may face in the eat-stop-eat protocol is the tendency to overeat on non-fasting days, sabotaging your weight loss efforts. After a fasting day, you may simply want to eat as much as you wish without caution to weight gain. This tendency is even raised if you have a risk of developing eating disorders.

Another challenge with the protocol is the tendency to ignore the protocol completely. The eat-stop-eat protocol has only one guideline, which you can utilize as you deem fit. If you are used to a more sophisticated dietary regimen, then you may find this protocol a bit too permissive, and this might cause you to discountenance it at some point.

Foods you can eat on the Eat-Stop-Eat protocol

The eat-stop-eat protocol does not put any food restrictions, just like most other intermittent fasting protocols. You may eat whatever you feel like eating on feasting days, even sodas and junk foods. However, in a bid to make this protocol more efficacious, it is highly recommended that you only eat a healthy, balanced diet constituted of lean proteins, veggies, complex carbs, and whole meals. On the reverse side, on fasting days, you can't take in foods that have calories. You may only take foods and drinks that don't contain calories, such as sugarless gum, coffee, tea, and water. Diet soda are also permissible if taken in moderation; of vital importance is that the drinks are sugarless. If you, however, prefer your drinks sweet, then you are allowed to add artificial sweeteners in your tea and coffee.

Foods to avoid on the Eat-Stop-Eat protocol

Just to reiterate, the eat-stop-eat protocol does not impose dietary restrictions of whatever kind on the dieter. As long as you adhere to your fasting schedule and restrict your calorie intake on fasting days to non-caloric drinks, there's no other thing to do. Again, as mentioned earlier, it is strongly recommended that you keep your junk food consumption at a minimum, so your weight loss efforts are not compromised.

How effective is the Eat-Stop-Eat protocol?

The eat-stop-eat protocol has the same level of efficacy in helping you lose weight as any other intermittent fasting protocol. As a primary benefit, this diet can allow your body to utilize stored fat. How it does this is by reducing and even exhausting the body's reserve of glucose and liver glycogen. In addition, it facilitates the production of the growth hormone, a hormone that can improve the body's fat-burning ability. Furthermore, this protocol is able to produce a big enough deficit in calories that your body requires to lose weight. One other factor that increases the efficacy of the eat-stop-eat protocol in relation to other intermittent fasting protocols is its simplicity. You only have to fast for a period of 24 hours twice a week. This is the only rule you need to observe. Being simple makes this protocol easier to stick to, and, therefore, more effective.

When you engage in the eat-stop-eat protocol, you can do some resistance or weight training to build and develop your muscle. Resistance or weight training is better than cardio and any other kinds of exercise that are exhaustive. It is not mandatory to exercise on fasting days, but you could put in place a few hours training schedule per week. Don't let it get too exhaustive; otherwise, you may feel the fast too severely.

Mistakes to avoid on the Eat-Stop-Eat protocol

There are two major mistakes you must try to avoid at all cost on the eat-stop-eat protocol. One of these potential mistakes is to overeat after completing a fast. As earlier stated, it might take your body some time to adjust to the new dietary system since you don't fast every day. Therefore, you may feel pangs of hunger on your fast days, together with general body weakness, fogginess, and headaches. If you are the working type, these symptoms may be even more severe. The sheer hunger you experience on your fast days may instigate you to binge-eat on feat days. When you binge-eat, the benefits you might have accrued the previous day would be canceled out by the excess food. Hence, your weight loss journey gets stalled. If you hope to prevent yourself from making this mistake, you must find effective methods of managing your hunger. According to Pilon, drinking drinks that don't contain calories can help reduce hunger. He also states that keeping yourself busy on fast days keeps you away from thinking about food. Another method you can use is to eat lots of proteins on the previous day before the fast so you can stay fuller for longer.

Another mistake you might make on this protocol is to be overly lenient with your fast schedule. One thing that makes the protocol attractive is that you can schedule your fast days whenever you like. However, the issue with this is that you may end up not fasting at all in a week because you keep postponing the fast days. To make sure that this doesn't happen, ensure to adhere to your schedule as strongly as possible. You may schedule your fast days to suit your professional and social life, but you must keep this behavior in check to avoid falling into the 'derailing' trap.

Is the Eat-Stop-Eat protocol healthy?

The eat-stop-eat protocol – as with most intermittent fasting protocols – is a healthy and safe diet protocol to indulge in. as far as science is concerned, the protocol does not pose any health hazards, nor does it have the potential to do so. However, just as you should do with all other types of intermittent fasting, if you are a pregnant woman, trying to get pregnant, or breastfeeding, then you should rethink starting on the protocol.

The restriction on food consumption on fast days may have certain effects on your hormones and may cause your body to behave in unexpected ways. It may also impact your body's process of producing breast milk. Also, if you are suffering from diabetes, endeavor to consult with your caregiver before you venture into the protocol. A drop in glucose levels may prove dangerous to your health. Lastly, if you have any eating disorder, have a history of or are at risk of developing one, then ensure that you check with your caregiver first. As earlier mentioned, intermittent fasting can induce binge eating. When this happens, your eating disorder may resurface, or your risk of developing one may get drastically increased.

While regular dietary regimens can become overly stressful and inconvenient by depriving you of your favorite foods, the eat-stop-eat protocol is aimed at removing stress from dieting while keeping you in touch with your most loved meals. The flexibility of the protocol makes it one of the most attractive dietary regimens to engage in and one that you should give a try. If you have tried some other intermittent fasting protocols and they haven't quite worked for you, then eat-stop-eat may be the thing for you. Even though it sounds more rigorous at first, protocol is actually one of the simplest and easiest weight loss dietary regimens out there.

Compared to the 5:2 protocol, for instance, you may feel that the 5:2 diet is easier to do because you get to eat 'something' on fast days. However, according to the experience of people who have tried it out, eating a little food on the 5:2 diet can make you hungrier you would be if you didn't eat anything at all. And if you're like such people as who feel hungrier when they eat small amounts of food, then you may find the eat-stop-eat diet easier to engage in.

D. The Warrior Protocol

The warrior protocol made its way into the diet world in 2001 when an ex-member of the Israeli Special Forces, Ori Hofmekler created it and espoused its working principles. It is another variety of intermittent fasting, which is a term used to describe a dietary pattern that involves an alternation between restricted and unrestricted feeding. The warrior diet is not predicated on any solid scientific findings, but rather on the feeding patterns of early humans, who were primarily warriors. These warriors consumed little food during the day because they were usually out hunting and ate most of their daily food at night. The diet, according to Hofmekler, is designed to bring out our innate survival instincts by putting the body through stress via reduced calorie intake.

The warrior protocol is fairly easy to understand: eat close to nothing for 20 hours and then eat as much as you like in the following 4 hours, specifically at night. While in the 20-hour fasting period, you are expected to eat little dairy products, boiled eggs, and raw fruits and veggies together with much non-calorie drinks. In the 4 hours of feasting, you may eat whatever you like. However, it is strongly recommended that you eat healthy, unprocessed foods so that your weight loss journey is not compromised. The warrior protocol can help burn fat, improve concentration, increase energy levels, and facilitate cellular repair. In addition, this protocol may improve mental health, reduce or prevent inflammation, and improve blood glucose level. It is a great protocol for people who want to eat as much food as they want while still losing weight.

Merits and Demerits of the Warrior Protocol

Some of the merits of the warrior diet include:

- **Aids weight loss:** Most intermittent fasting protocols have been associated with weight loss. The warrior diet is not exempt from this benefit. Fasting on alternate days on a regular basis has been proved to help people struggling with weight issues shed body fat.
- **Improved blood sugar levels:** The warrior diet in particular – and fasting in general – helps improve insulin sensitivity, thereby improving blood sugar level. However, for you to enjoy this benefit, you must cut down on your carbs intake during the feeding period.
- **May be effective against inflammation:** Inflammation is one of the commonest causes of diseases, such as cardiovascular diseases, diabetes, bowel anomalies, and certain cancers. Research in the area of intermittent fasting has proved that fasting can help kick against inflammation.
- **May reduce the risk for certain cognitive diseases:** Studies on animals have concluded that intermittent fasting can help prolong the onset of degenerative diseases, such as Alzheimer's disease. However, there is a dearth of research in the area, and more studies are going to be needed to verify this claim.

The warrior protocol is not without its own flaws. Here are some of its demerits:

- **It may be difficult to adhere to:** While out hunter-gatherer ancestors might have been able to go 20 hours without much food, which is clearly not in the norm of the contemporary world. And our bodies have not been conditioned to that kind of dietary pattern. It is difficult to fast for 20 hours a day and might come with side effects such as headaches, hunger pangs, and cravings.
- **It may trigger bingeing:** The warrior protocol does allow a dieter to eat for 4 hours in every 24. Due to the hunger pangs, the dieter might have endured during the fasting

window, and they may binge heavily in the feasting window. In addition, you may have obsessive thoughts about eating during fasting.

- **It may not be suitable for certain groups of people:** Women who are breastfeeding or pregnant may not be able to follow the warrior diet. People with diabetes may not be able to stay off sources of glucose for as long as 20 hours. For these people, the warrior protocol is deemed inappropriate.
- **Has potential adverse effects:** Not eating for 20 hours on end may cause you to be exposed to certain side effects including fogginess, fatigue, mood swings, anxiety, lightheadedness, hormonal anomalies, and severe stress.
- **Deficiencies of nutrients:** You are permitted to eat for only 4 hours out of possible 24; therefore, you may not be able to consume the appropriate amounts of nutrients your body requires. This is usually the case when a dieter focuses heavily on consuming carbs.

What to Eat on the Warrior Protocol

The warrior protocol does not impose any restrictions on what to eat during the 4-hour feasting window. It, however, recommends that you eat healthy, non-processed, whole meals, as they can aid your weight loss endeavor. Here are some foods you should try to consume on the warrior diet:

- **Fruits and veggies:** It is highly recommended that you consume some fruits and veggies on a daily basis in order to ensure that your body gets the vital minerals and vitamins it requires to perform optimally.
- **Grains:** Eat whole-grain food, including wheat bread, rice, quinoa, oatmeal, and bulgur. These are all great additions that you can fuel up from in the feasting phase.
- **Dairy:** The warrior diet strongly recommends consuming dairy products, particularly raw and full-fat dairy foods, like yogurt, raw milk, and cheese.
- **Protein:** Protein-containing foods are advised for people on the warrior protocol. Protein is crucial for building and developing muscle, which in itself is a goal of the warrior protocol.
- **Beverages:** It is permitted to consume beverages that don't contain calories during the fasting period, such as coffee, tea, and water. You can consume any beverage during the feasting phase.

What Not to Eat on the Warrior Protocol

Again, the warrior protocol does not explicitly restrict dieters from consuming any kinds of food. However, in order to maximize the outcome of the diet, you should only eat healthy foods and shun unhealthy ones. Here are certain food types you should consider abstaining from on the warrior protocol:

- **Sugar-containing processed products:** Sugary foods in packs have been heavily linked with the development of many chronic illnesses, such as diabetes and certain bowel abnormalities. Ensure that you keep your processed sugar consumption to a bare minimum.

- **Salty processed products:** Although you may feel that this group of foods is healthier than sugary foods, salty processed foods might be as damning to your blood sugar and overall health. If you feel like eating something crunchy, give veggies with hummus a try. You may also opt to prepare your own snacks at home.
- **Sugary beverages:** Consumption of sodas, energy-boosting drinks, and juice containing sugar should be kept at a bare minimum. Sugar-containing beverages are common causes of weight gain and illness.

When you should Schedule your Fasting and Feasting

As with many intermittent fasting protocols, timing is a key component of the warrior protocol. The entire protocol is founded on the idea that a long duration of fasting and a short period of feasting can result in improved health and body composition. During the fasting phase of the protocol, you are encouraged to eat only foods that have minimal to no calories, particularly dairy foods, boiled eggs, and raw fruits and veggies. You may also choose to take drinks that don't contain calories, such as coffee and water. You may eat as you wish during the feasting window of 4 hours. When to schedule these 4 hours is entirely left to your personal preference. However, it is common practice for people to reserve their feasting for evening hours.

Dos and Don'ts while on the Warrior Protocol

If you want to optimize the warrior protocol, then you should endeavor to adhere to the following guidelines.

- **DON'T** count your calories: One of the many benefits of the warrior protocol and indeed of most intermittent fasting protocols is that you don't have to count calories or monitor closely the foods that you eat. As long as you keep to the plan, nothing else needs to be done.
- **DO** avoid consuming processed foods: avoid eating processed or packaged foods. Instead, shift to focus to ingesting whole, organic foods like salads on a regular basis.
- **DON'T** shy away from drinking water: Drinking lots of water is a diet hack – it can fill you up, thereby alleviating hunger, has inherent health benefits, and does not come with calories. Make water a close companion of yours on the protocol.
- **DO** vary your diet: Eat a wide range of nutrients if you want your body to gain all of the nutrients it requires. This should include fruits and vegetables alongside animal-based proteins and grains.
- **DON'T** start on the warrior protocol if you suffer from an eating disorder: The warrior protocol recommends eating large amounts of food during the 4-hour eating window. This could be detrimental to your health if you already have an eating disorder or have the risk factors for developing one.
- **DO** ingest a multivitamin: Eating a multivitamin on a daily basis in collaboration with your varied daily diet can serve as much needed insurance.

CHAPTER 3

INTERMITTENT FASTING VS STARVATION

Intermittent fasting is based on the idea that keeping food away for a period of time can make you lose weight, and, training in such a state can make your build lean muscle. However, several people have raised doubts as to whether intermittent fasting can indeed cause your body to go into starvation mode. This has been a heated issue over the last years and continues to be a major factor hindering some people from embarking on intermittent fasting. The case of the risk of starvation while fasting is important because, according to certain sources, your body starts to deplete its protein stores and save fat while in the starvation mode. This is sharply opposed to what anyone engaging in intermittent fasting would want.

Before we explain how starvation works and whether or not your body can be plunged into starvation mode by fasting, we must first discuss what starvation really is. So, what exactly is the starvation mode, and why does it matter?

Starvation mode is activated if your body is starved of essential nutrients for a prolonged period of time. In starvation mode, your body, not knowing what else to do, starts to eat up some of its protein content (particularly those in the muscles) ad a way of producing the energy it requires for carrying out basic internal activities. The starvation mode is dangerous because it detracts from your wellbeing. There are two kinds of starvation: short-term starvation and long-term starvation.

Short-term starvation is basically depriving your body of nutrients for a short period of time. In essence, it is not even starvation. It does not have any lasting effects and does not change your basal metabolic rate, which is the number of calories your body burns while at rest. It's just a few hours of not eating, something that the world starvation does not truly describe.

Long-term starvation, on the other hand, is a situation where you starve your body of nutrients for a long period of time. This is the real starvation, and the one people resort to when they want to lose weight. Weight is one of the factors the body's basal metabolic rate. So when you lose weight through starvation, the basal metabolic rate gradually decreases. This is an outcome of weight loss that cannot be avoided.

Difference between Calorie Restriction, Fasting, and Starvation

There is a difference between Calorie restriction, fasting, and starvation.

Starvation is a situation of grave deficiency in nutrient intake. During starvation, the body does not have access to vital nutrients and, therefore, it starts to cannibalize on its internal organs for energy. Starvation is a gradual process in which the body slowly wastes away by eating up its proteins and storing up fat. This is the reason for the skinny-fat appearance of people who are starving. One of the signs of starvation is the bloated stomach appearance or kwashiorkor, that results from low protein consumption, even in the face of adequate carb ingestion.

Calorie restriction is limiting calorie intake without throwing the body into a malnourished state. If you're on a calorie restriction regimen, what you're doing is basically reducing the number of calories you consume while maintaining the minimum energy requirements your body requires to function optimally. This helps to shed some of your stored fat, reduce basal metabolic rate, improve the functioning of certain hormones, and facilitate gluconeogenesis. The major difference between Calorie restriction and starvation is, during calorie restriction, your body still gets the number of calories it needs to perform its basic internal activities. In essence, you're still fulfilling your body's energy demands, although the energy demands may have been modified to adapt to the nutrients your body gets.

Fasting is basically putting a stop to calorie consumption. During fasting, your body still gets the energy it needs by resorting to ketosis – using up stored fat to fulfill its energy needs. There is no danger that you might lack the micronutrients you need when you're fasting because your body has already stored up a number of micronutrients it can use throughout the fasting period.

Signs your Body is in Starvation Mode

Here are some signs to watch out for, which can signal that your body has gone into starvation mode:

- **You always feel hungry:** It is normal to feel hungry while fasting; this is a small tradeoff for the greater good that is losing weight. However, if you start to feel hungry all the time and binge whenever you have the slightest chance, then there is a deep change going on in your system. Hunger is regulated by two hormones – leptin, which makes you feel full; ghrelin, which makes you feel hunger. Leptin is produced from the body's fat cells, and it is logical that leptin levels go down as you lose fat. This, you feel hungrier. But then, studies have shown that leptin levels can drastically decrease due to a severe deficiency in calorie intake, notwithstanding if weight is lost.
- **There is a general feeling of lethargy:** Starvation mode makes you feel so lethargic that you are not able to perform the activities you normally perform. In this case, activities such as getting out of bed and using the stairs start to seem like Herculean tasks to you, and you simply want to sleep all day instead.
- **Your weight loss stalls:** If you are getting in more exercise while eating the same calories but failing to lose weight, your body may have entered starvation mode. Not losing weight for a number of days is not something to worry about. However, if you don't lose weight for a few weeks consecutively and have reached your minimal calorie intake, then you may be in starvation mode.
- **You get cold:** Research has proved that restricting calorie intake for a long period of time can reduce the body's core temperature. If you find yourself getting cold always, even in warm conditions, you may be in starvation mode.

How to Avoid Getting into Starvation Mode

The following are tips to help you avoid getting into starvation mode.

- Ensure you remain in fasting for at least 16 hours a day on fasting days. This would help to make your body resort to ketosis.
- Avoid consuming foods that contain calories during the fasting period. Everything that contains calories can slow down autophagy or inhibit it.
- Take foods such as coffee and green tea while in the fasting window. These help to boost autophagy and promote ketosis. Make sure you don't add any sweeteners, sugar, oils, or milk in the drinks, as they can get your body out of the fasted state.
- Drink lots of salted water. Adding sodium and magnesium salts in your drinking water can help replenish your electrolytes and prevent cramps.
- Engage more in dry fasting than regular fasting. Dry fasting can get your body in ketosis quicker.
- Watch what you eat in your feasting windows. Eat foods that can maintain your blood sugar levels while keeping your insulin levels in check. Add ginger and turmeric to your diet alongside fats, carbs, and proteins.

How to get your Body out of Starvation Mode

The best thing to do in your intermittent fasting journey is to avoid getting into starvation mode at all cost. If you do get into starvation mode, however, here are some tips to help you get your body out of it:

- **Eat more calories:** The first step to take while in starvation mode is to eat more calories. By eating more calories, you bridge the calorie deficit that got you into the situation in the first place.
- **Increase your protein intake:** Proteins take a lot of energy to get digested. Adding more proteins to your diet raises your basal metabolic rate and promotes lean muscle gain.
- **Take a break:** Sometimes, you need to take a break from your fasting regimen to allow your body some respite. If you're already in starvation mode, there's little progress you can make going forward.

Starvation mode is a long-term impact of calorie restriction that results from a severe deficiency in nutrient intake. It does not result from limiting calorie intake for a few days or weeks, and, therefore, is not likely to happen while you're on intermittent fasting. All you have to do is consume enough macro and micronutrients, drink lots of water, and exercise at the appropriate times, and your weight loss endeavor will be well on track.

CHAPTER 4

INTERMITTENT FASTING WITH WORKOUTS

Intermittent fasting has been able to garner as much following as it now has due to many reasons, one of which is its flexibility and simplicity. There are many different intermittent fasting protocols to choose from, and each of them comes with specific instructions as to how to schedule the feasting and fasting periods. These protocols vary in this aspect, and the variation is important to people willing to try intermittent fasting, and they have a wealth of options to choose from. However, concerns have been raised about whether or not exercising is indeed good for the body during fasting. And these concerns seemingly keep on growing.

If you are wondering whether you can work out while fasting or not, then the simple answer you are looking for is "yes." But, of course, you are not looking for a simple answer. Chances are, you would like to know how exercising in a fasted state affects your health and the overall outcome of your intermittent fasting regimen. The truth is, as is the case with many other things, there are pros and cons to working out during fasting.

There are studies that have associated working out during fasting with body chemistry and certain metabolic activities concerning insulin sensitivity and blood sugar levels. There are also studies that support exercising just after eating a meal before the meal has had the time to get digested or absorbed. This routine is particularly helpful to people with a sort of metabolic disorder or people suffering from diabetes.

One of the many benefits of intermittent fasting is that, while fasting, the body's deposited of glycogen get depleted, thereby leading to weight loss gain through fat-burning. Therefore, working out can make you burn fat, as the body uses stored fat as fuel to support itself. This assertion is backed by scientific studies. There are studies that have come out to counter this assertion; however, by staying that fasting on an empty stomach does not help you lose more fat. A particularly crucial downside of working out while fasting is that your body may start to use protein (such as that of muscle) to fuel its activities. In addition to the fact that depleting your muscle to fuel workouts is counterintuitive, you may not be able to perform as much as you would if, for instance, the source of energy came from carbs or fats. Furthermore, metabolism may get slowed in this entire process, further compromising your muscle gain endeavor.

Overall, working out in a fasted state is a dicey situation: yes, you may lose more fat, but if done over a long period of time, your metabolism could get impeded. You may not be able to perform as much as you would like, and may not be able to build muscle. There are upsides and downsides to consider. The benefit of fasted workout depends on a lot of factors, such as your age, physical health condition, level of fitness, lifestyle, and fasting goals. If you are a professional athlete, then fasted training may not be appropriate for you. For people who do a lot of workouts, intermittent fasting may not be a good fit.

Working out while fasting can exert a lot of stress on your metabolic and physical systems, and for you to support your workout while maintaining muscle mass, you need to consume lots of calories in meals taken strategically throughout the day. Fasted working depends heavily on your individual body requirements and functioning. It is an individual thing, and there is no one answer that is suitable for everyone.

If you have elected to work out while on an intermittent fasting protocol, then there are certain guidelines you should adhere to. Here they are:

- **Get your timing right:** According to experts, timing either to work out before, during, or after the feasting window is key to the outcome of the workout and of the entire intermittent fasting protocol you are on. Lean gains is a protocol that particular emphasizes training or working out while in a fasted state. Whether you work out before, during, or after the feasting window would depend on your personal preference entirely. If you enjoy working out on an empty stomach, then you should consider working out before the feasting window. If you don't like to work out on an empty stomach, then you should work out during the feasting window, when you can capitalize on post-workout vitamins, minerals, and macronutrients in meals. If you want better performance and recovery, then it is recommended that you schedule your workout during the feasting window. Working out after the feasting period is ideally suited to individuals who enjoy training after feeding or who do not have the time to exercise before or during the feasting window.
- **Tailor your choice of workout to suit your macronutrients:** It is vital that you observe the micronutrients you ingest before working out and those you consume later on, and try to match your choice of workout to the type of micronutrients you take. For example, if you wish to engage in strength workouts, the eating lots of carbs on the workout day would help. You should reserve cardio workouts for low-carb days.
- **Eat appropriate meals after working out in order to maintain or build muscle mass:** A safe and healthy way to exercise during fasting is to schedule your workouts such that you consume essential nutrients after working out. If your workouts are rife with lifting heavy weights, then you must ingest enough proteins after your training, in order to make room for regeneration. As a general rule, ensure to eat carbs and about 15-20 grams of protein within 30 minutes after working out.
- **Keep your body in a hydrated state:** You must remember to drinks lots of water to keep yourself hydrated while fasting and especially while engaged in workouts.
- **Maintain a high electrolyte level:** Of you are looking for an alternative to water as a source of hydration, then coconut water is a good fit for you. Coconut water is good as a hydrating agent, taste good, and is filled with electrolytes. What's more, it is low in calories, so it doesn't interfere greatly with your fasting protocol. You must avoid drinking sodas and sports drinks that have high sugar content.
- **Keep intensity low at first:** If you are new to exercising while fasting, then it is not logical or healthy to start off by pushing yourself too hard. Get some low-intensity workouts under your belt in the first few days or weeks, and then grow into it gradually.
- **Take the type of protocol you're on into consideration:** The type of intermittent fasting protocol you're on can affect your workout regimen. If you are on the 24-hour fast, for instance, then the intensity of your workout should be lower than if you are on the 16-hour fasting protocol. Consider doing low-intensity training if you're on a physically demanding fasting protocol, like walking and restorative yoga.

- **Pay close attention to your body:** It is important that you observe your body and look out for signs that your workout regimen is getting out of hand. If you're starting to feel weak and dizzy, know that your body may be trying to tell you that it is dehydrated or low on glucose. If this happens, then reach for a carbohydrate-electrolyte drink immediately and then eat a balanced diet later on.
- **Keep your protein consumption on a high wine feasting:** If you are looking to get serious about building muscle mass, then you're going to be needing lots of proteins before and after every strength training. While taking a snack before working out can help your body fuel up, a protein intensive meal can do a lot for muscle synthesis both after your workout (when your muscles are most likely to crave amino acids for muscle repair and development) and throughout your day. In order to optimize the process of muscle development, you must endeavor to take about 20-30 grams of protein every 3 to 4 hours during the day and right after training, according to the Academy of Nutrition and Dietetics. To make things better, sandwich your strength training between two meals, so your body can benefit from two large bouts of nutrients.
- **Take advantage of snacks:** Some intermittent fasting protocols permit eating snacks as part of meal plans. You must use this flexibility to your advantage. Consuming a snack few hours (or a couple of hours, if you are more likely to suffer from low blood sugar) before working out can ensure that you don't lack the essential nutrients your body requires to perform at optimum. Your aim should be a meal that contains both quick-acting carbs and blood glucose-regulating proteins.

Is it possible to build muscle while on intermittent fasting?

It is possible to build muscle mass while on intermittent fasting. All you have to do is nourish your body with the nutrients it requires to function optimally. The most important of these nutrients are macronutrients, such as protein and carbs. In addition to these, you should take dietary supplements like BCAA, which can further boost your energy levels and improve metabolism.

When to stop working out

As earlier stated, when it comes to exercising while fasting, it is important that you pay close attention to your body and how it reacts. A major turn off in fasted training is extremely low blood glucose levels that can trigger reactions like dizziness and even fainting. For starters, you must assess what your first meal of the day is and how it sits well with your intended workout regimen. While you should eat carbs together with proteins and fats on a regular diet, you should eat more complex carbs during the feasting window of a fasted training day. Failure to do this could potentially increase your chances of developing an injury or experiencing side effects, some of which have been discussed earlier.

The primary purpose of most intermittent fasting protocols is to make the body shed weight by subjecting it to calorie restriction. While you may have a secondary purpose in addition to this, you must always bear in mind that whatever you do, you don't want to compromise the primary purpose of your intermittent fasting regimen. Training while fasting is a good way to further shed weight while maintaining and possibly building muscle mass. However, you must pay attention to certain markers that may signal that your body cannot cope with the training regimen while fasting. A rule of thumb is to schedule your fasted training for after one meal and before another, as this ensures that your body is treated to the right amounts of nutrients it requires. As for the meals, keep them filled with essential nutrients and strengthen them with snacks when necessary. In addition, there are supplements you can take to boost your metabolism and energy levels. Endeavor to use these supplements judiciously.

CHAPTER 5

EATING RULES

Most, if not all, intermittent fasting protocols do not place restrictions on the sort of food to eat. They don't draw distinct lines as to what to eat and what not to eat during either the fasting or the feasting periods. However, intermittent fasting protocols do not encourage or promote unhealthy eating habits. You can't simply eat whatever you like because there are no restrictions on what to eat. You must endeavor to eat healthy foods, drinks, and snacks. That is the best way to gain maximum benefit from your intermittent fasting struggle. It is strongly recommended that you speak with a nutrition expert before you make any wholesale changes to your diet, as your body might react to the alterations you make in unexpected ways.

If you want to maximize the efficacy of intermittent fasting, whether it is weight loss or muscle gain, or a combination of both that is your goal, you must eat balanced diets throughout the fasting protocol you're on. Avoid taking foods like junk and sugary, processed foods, and stick instead to whole meals, vegetables, fruits, and proteins. The following are recommended foods to eat while on an intermittent fasting protocol.

- **Water:** This is a no-brainer. Water is a vital component of our bodies and one that our cells need to perform optimally. You should endeavor to stay hydrated by drinking lots of water during feasting and fasting periods, as your system depends on it for survival and performance. The amount of water you should drink is not a fixed number; it varies from person to person and from circumstance to circumstance. A good way to check if you are drinking enough water is to observe the color of your urine. If you are properly hydrated, your urine would have a pale yellow color. If your urine has a dark yellow color, it might be indicative of the fact that you are dehydrated. Dehydrated states often lead to headaches, dizziness, and lightheadedness. If you add this to the fact that you are not getting enough food, then you may as well be preparing for a disaster. If you can't bat to drink plain water all day long, then you could 'spice' it up by adding a bit of lemon juice, cucumber, or mint leaves to your water before drinking. This is a life hack.
- **Avocado:** It may seem a counteractive thing to eat high-calorie foods while trying to shed weight, but avocado is incredibly satiating, thanks to the monounsaturated fats it contains. As a hack, you could add half avocado to your during feasting periods. Doing so can make you feel fuller for hours more than you would if you didn't consume the green gem.
- **Fish:** There is a good reason why experts advise that you add some ounces of fish to your meal every week. Fish is rich in healthy proteins and fats and is a reserve of vitamin D. Fish is a great addition to your diet, particularly if you're only allowed to eat small amounts of food (like during the fasting period). Fish is known as "brain food "; hence, it helps to prevent certain cognitive drops that are associated with fasting.
- **Cruciferous vegetables:** Vegetables like broccoli, cauliflower, and Brussels sprouts are rich in fiber. It is recommended that you eat lots of fiber when you have to restrict your calorie intake, as they can help prevent constipation and maintain regularity. Fibers have been proven to make you feel full, which is an invaluable addition for when you have to

fast for a long stretch of time. Imagine fasting for 16 hours straight! You would need anything that can keep you feeling full.

- **Potatoes:** This may come as a shock addition, but you must remember that some white foods are good. As you probably know, and as studies have found, potatoes are some of the most filling foods out there. This is not to say you should consume French fries and potato chips, as these can be detrimental to weight. You should rather eat potatoes incorporated into a healthy diet.
- **Legumes and beans:** Beans may just be the best friend you are looking for in your intermittent fasting journey. Beans and legumes are carbs that are low in calories, which can help boost your energy levels to perform activities. Foods such as black beans and chickpeas have been found to help reduce weight, even without the intervention of a dietary protocol.
- **Probiotics:** There is nothing your gut loves more than consistency when it comes to dieting. And nothing it hates more than having to stay hungry. When your gut is sad, you experience symptoms like constipation and other bowel irregularities. To combat this, make sure to include foods that are rich in probiotics, such as Kefir and Kraut, to your daily meal plan.
- **Berries:** While berries may be your favorite addition to smoothies, they may also be your favorite companions on the intermittent fasting journey because they are rich in essential nutrients. A cup of strawberries, for instance, contains about the daily requirement of vitamin C, which helps to boost immunity. Although not concrete yet, there are studies suggesting that people who ingest flavonoids in foods containing them, such as blueberries and strawberries, showed an improvement in body mass index compared to people who didn't.
- **Eggs:** Eggs are undisputed sources of proteins that get cooked in minutes. If your interest is to keep full for as long as possible and build muscle mass, then you should consider making eggs a part of your diet. Eggs have been found to keep you fuller than a bagel would.
- **Nuts:** Although nuts might contain more calories than many junk foods, they possess good fat, which most junk foods do not contain. According to studies, the polyunsaturated fat in walnuts can modify the physiology of hunger and satiety.
- **Whole grains:** It might seem as though eating carbs while on a diet is a misfit. But that is not always the case. True whole-grain meals contain proteins and fiber, substances that can keep you feeling full for longer. According to research, eating whole grains can do a lot more for your metabolism than eating refined grains. So, eat much whole grain foods as part of your diet, including millet, sorghum, freekeh, and bulgur.
- **Coffee:** One substance that has been repeatedly mentioned in the intermittent fasting protocols mentioned in this book is coffee. Newbies often get confused as to whether coffee may break their fast. But you don't need to worry at all; coffee is allowed on most intermittent fasting protocols. Coffee, when nothing else is added into it, is essentially calorie-free, so you can have it within or outside the limits of a fasting window. However, coffee becomes restricted too if certain substances have been added to it, like creamers and

flavorings. Creamed or flavored coffee can no longer be taken in the fasting period, so be cautious of how you doctor your coffee.

- **Lentils:** Lentils are nutritional commandos. You can get as much as 30 percent of your daily fiber requirements in half a cup of lentils. Lentils also contain good amounts of iron (contains about 15 percent of your daily iron needs), which is a vital supplement for fasting women who are still active.
- **Seitan**: Some experts have stressed the fact that animal-based proteins should be taken cautiously if one intends to prolong longevity. Seitan is a plant-based protein that has an inherent capacity to increase life span. Seitan can be baked, battered, or used with sauce.
- **Hummus:** Hummus is yet another plant-based protein substitute. If you wish to make your own hummus, then remember to add lots of garlic and tahini to it.
- **Wild-caught salmon:** Salmons are rich in certain substances called omega-3 fatty acids, which can help boost the brain. These substances are EPA and DHA.
- **Soybeans:** There is literally no further need to state why you should eat soybeans. Reasons abound as to why you should incorporate this food into your diet. Soybeans contain isoflavones, substances that have been proved to help prevent UVB-induced damage to cells as well as decrease aging.
- **Multivitamins:** One of the basic principles of intermittent fasting and why it promises to be effective for weight loss lies in the fact that fasting makes you eat less, and, therefore, gives your body less opportunity to gain weight. This deficit in food intake can lead to your body having fewer nutrients than it needs. Having multivitamin as part of your daily diet plan can help ensure that you don't lack the essential vitamins your body requires.
- **Smoothies:** If taking a multivitamin does not quite cut it for you, then you could supplement your diet with a homemade smoothie filled with veggies and fruits. Smoothies offer you a way to have a mix of many different kinds of food containing different sorts of nutrients.
- **Milk fortified with vitamin D:** The required calcium intake for an adult is 1 gram per day, equivalent to 3 cups of milk. When your diet is restricted, you get fewer opportunities to take as much calcium ad you need. That's why you must seize every opportunity to take more calcium. Milk fortified with vitamin D gives the body a chance to absorb more vitamin D and thus helps keep your bones strong. If you want to increase your calcium intake, simply add milk to your cereals or take milk with your meals. However, if you don't fancy dairy products, then you could take substitutes such as kale and tofu.
- **Papaya:** The effects of fasting may start to hit home towards the end of the fasting period, especially if you are new to intermittent fasting. Hunger pangs may you lead to overeating when your feasting window finally open, leaving you feeling lethargic. Papaya has an ability to break down proteins through its enzyme papain, and eating papaya as part of your meal can help your digestion and prevent bloating.
- **Ghee:** Ghee is simply clarified butter. Because it had a high smoke point, it can replace your regular cooking oil, especially when you're making hot fries.
- **Branch chain amino acid (BCAA) supplement:** BCAA is a supplement that can help with muscle development, especially during fasted training. Taking BCAA supplement is

stressed in the lean gains protocol, which encourages exercising during the fasting period. However, the supplement can be consumed any time in the day, whether you are fasting or not, as it helps prevent muscle loss. Most of this supplement is produced from duck feathers, so it is a no-go-area if you are a vegan.

Although the intermittent fasting protocols mentioned in this book do not place restrictions upon what to eat or what not to, it is imperative that you do yourself a favor by eating only healthy foods that can maximize the outcome of your intermittent fasting endeavor. Use the details provided here as not instructions but guidelines, tips, and tricks to help you make the best out of whatever intermittent fasting protocol you have chosen to follow.

CHAPTER 6

SIDE EFFECTS OF INTERMITTENT FASTING

Intermittent fasting is one of the healthiest and trendiest ways to deal with the issues of weight gain at the moment. There are many protocols to follow in the intermittent fasting world, and most, if not all, of them, have two periods of time – a feeding period when you can eat freely and a fasting period when you are to restrict eating or calorie intake.

Logic and scientific studies have backed intermittent fasting as a healthy way to lose fat and build muscle tissue both in the short term and the long term. Apart from helping you lose weight, intermittent fasting has also been found to help the body fend off certain diseases conditions and prevent others from developing. The diseases that intermittent fasting can help keep at bay include Alzheimer's disease, bowel diseases, and even cancer. Some people have even asserted that intermittent fasting can help initiate cellular repair and prolong life. While all of these assertions have scientific backing, some of the scientific studies done in support of these assertions have been done on animals, leaving only a few human studies. Even the studies on humans are mostly short-term studies lasting only a few months. This issue is pointed out by Howard Steiger, a psychiatry professor at McGill University, who said that there is a dearth of long-term studies backing the asserted benefits of intermittent fasting.

On the flip side, intermittent fasting has not been shown by scientific studies to be harmful to people who are of sound health, notwithstanding if they have normal weight, are overweight, or are obese. So, it is a matter of two ends – while it cannot be stressed that intermittent fasting is harmful, the reverse cannot be supported with tangible scientific evidence. Therefore, if you do wish to embark on any intermittent fasting protocol, then you must do so with caution and in the knowledge that you are not suffering from any condition that may react negatively to intermittent fasting.

Before you decide to start on intermittent fasting, you must have an honest conversation with your caregiver. This should be done in all cases and especially if you have risk factors for developing certain health anomalies. On a general note, if you are 65 or older, whether you feel healthy or not, make sure to have that conversation with your physician. If you are on any sort of medication, this consultation would also hold true for you and importantly so. This is so because medications are usually hinged on regular diets. And intermittent fasting is anything but regular. Another group of people that must be wary of venturing into intermittent fasting is that of heavy equipment handling. If you are a driver or in charge of handling heavy machinery, then intermittent fasting may be inappropriate for you. You may feel lightheaded or dizzy while fasting – symptoms that can be detrimental to your work life.

People who are in need of high calories are not encouraged to fast. These people include individuals younger than 18, underweight people, and pregnant and breastfeeding women, according to experts. It is also recommended that you not fast if you have diabetes or are at risk of developing it since blood glucose levels are at risk of going below healthy levels during fasting. Also, if you have risk factors for any eating disorders, such as binge eating disorder, you shouldn't do intermittent fasting. Risk factors to watch out for are family members that have an eating disorder, mood swings, or perfectionism. Calorie restriction for a long stretch of time can result in the development of an eating disorder if you already possess risk factors.

Despite the multitudes of benefits that can be obtained from intermittent fasting, it must be said that intermittent fasting has its own cons. These cons come by way of side effects accompanying the feasting and fasting regimens designed to be followed by dieters. Here are some of the side effects of intermittent fasting:

- **You may feel terribly hungry:** If you are used to eating constantly, then you may feel terrible hunger pangs during the fasting hours of an intermittent fasting protocol. However, there may be a way to help yourself out and keep hunger in check. While fasting, keep yourself from looking at, smelling, or having thoughts about food. All of these can act as triggers in the release of stomach acid that makes you feel hungry, according to Yuan-Xiang Pan, a University of Illinois associate professor of nutrition. Pan suggests engaging in activities that get your mind off the thoughts of food, such as reading a book or any other mentally tasking activity. He particularly discourages sitting in front of the TV as it is a sedentary thing to do and can cause food thoughts to crawl into your mind. If you need to take in something, consider taking water, coffee, or sugarless tea, says Pan.

  What is even better than having to deal with hunger pangs is preventing it altogether. You can keep hunger out by eating a balanced diet that keeps you feeling fuller for longer. This means you must direct your focus to fiber, proteins, and healthy fats, as they are effective in keeping hunger away.

  According to experts, it is recommended that you begin your intermittent fasting journey slow and gradually growing into it. Pick a protocol that resonates with your needs and personal preferences and try it out for a week. This way, you can evaluate how well you do and know whether to continue on it or try out another protocol. There are many intermittent fasting protocols to choose from – the lean gains, fast diet, eat-stop-eat, and warrior diet, among others – all of which have their own unique requirements and guidelines. Get to know which works for you. If you are trying out intermittent fasting for the first time, then, rather than abstaining from eating altogether, start by cutting your calories in half and see how well you do.

- **There is danger of over-eating:** The non-fasting days of most intermittent fasting protocols are days on which you can eat whatever you want, whenever you want, and however, you want. The bad news is, if you overeat on your feasting days, your net calorie intake may then be higher than what it would be on a normal day. In summary, your efforts at losing weight may be compromised. On the other hand, fasting for long periods of time may induce binge-eating. In fact, fasting is a major trigger of binge-eating and has been found to cause bingeing in people with risk factors.

- **Intermittent fasting may cause dehydration:** Intermittent fasting has been associated with dehydration. This is so because not eating can cause you not to drink as well. You must endure to remain adequately hydrated while fasting by taking lots of fluids.

- **You may get tired:** Intermittent fasting can cause you to feel groggy, especially if you are new to the intermittent fasting world. While fasting, your body runs on less 'fuel' than normal, and since fasting can increase stress, your sleep patterns may also get disrupted. Try engaging in stress-relieving exercises, such as meditation and listening to music. If you already have a training or fitness schedule in place, then schedule your training for eating hours. By so doing, you help yourself conserve energy. You also avoid having an increased risk of sustaining an injury, which may occur when you train while fasting.

- **Irritability:** appetite and moods are governed by the same biochemistry. Your nutrient intake can affect how certain neurotransmitters – such as dopamine and serotonin – work. These neurotransmitters can have a role in disorders like anxiety and depression. This means that disruptions in your dietary habits can affect your mood as well. A way to keep this in check is to adhere to a balanced diet and eating foods that can help keep you full for longer. Furthermore, you must ensure to get enough sleep, as it is linked to mood.

- **Cravings:** Intermittent fasting can cause you to have cravings for food, since they restrict you from eating whatever you want, whenever you want. For instance, if you are asked to stop eating a certain fruit forever, chances are, all you would want to eat is that fruit. Intermittent fasting exposes you to long periods of time without ingesting food. Therefore, there is a great chance that all you'd want to do while fasting is to eat some food. This is how cravings set in. you may crave mostly sugary drinks and carbs because your body is in a severe need of glucose. Instead of budge to your cravings, you should do everything you can to stop food thoughts in their tracks. Ensure to satisfy your cravings during the feasting window.

- **Headaches:** A your system is still trying to adjust to the new dietary pattern, side effects of fasting may start to kick in. A common side effect of intermittent fasting is headache. According to experts, dehydration may be one of the factors that cause headaches during fasting. Therefore, you must endeavor to drink lots of fluid when you are fasting. In addition, lowered blood glucose levels may also cause headaches, alongside certain hormones released by your brain during the fasting period. Your body should adapt to your new dietary patterns as time goes on and all should be well in time.

- **Low energy levels:** Due to the fasting regimen, your body would get low on energy as it no longer gets as many nutrients to produce energy as it normally does. So, you may feel a little sluggish during fasting, especially in the first few weeks. To combat this, try to conserve energy as much as possible while fasting, and keep your day stress-free. You shouldn't engage in workouts deep into the fasting period when you are weak, and if you must do some sort of exercise, consider engaging in walking or yoga.

- **Heartburn, constipation, and bloating:** Your stomach produces hydrochloric acid, which helps it to digest eaten food. So while fasting, you may have heartburn as a result of the action of that acid. Heartburn symptoms vary from person to person. Some people may experience only mild discomfort, while some others may experience full-blown pain. Given time, this side effect should vanish, so all you have to do is keep taking water and avoid foods that can worsen your heartburn, such as spicy foods. If your heartburn does not disappear after some time, consider seeing a physician. A solution to the problem of constipation is to take more water, especially when thirsty. Furthermore, take some magnesium citrate to assist in hydrating your bowel and aiding peristalsis (bowel motion).

- **Bathroom trips:** Fasting can make you drink more water than you would on a normal day. Drinking more water means you have a greater need to visit the bathroom. You might find yourself going to the bathroom as many as twice in an hour. As trivial as this seems, it may be well discomforting, especially if you are doing something that requires you to remain at a spot for a period of time. There may be no way around this other than remaining as close to the bathroom as possible.
- **Intermittent fasting can disrupt your sleep pattern:** Studies have shown that intermittent fasting can disrupt your Rapid Eye Movement (REM) sleep, which is vital to memory, learning capacity, and mood.
- **Decreased levels of alertness and awareness:** Some people, including Twitter CEO Jack Dorsey, have claimed that fasting improves their focus and alertness. However, these claims have been rubbished by nutrition experts, who say this extra focus and alertness one feels while fasting is due to the lack of food that throws the brain into starvation mode. Feeling more focused and alert while fasting is a way your brain tells you it is in need of food, which makes fasting counterproductive for focus and alertness. In the long term, you may feel less focused and alert because your body does not have enough calories to perform optimally.
- **Feeling of stress:** Intermittent fasting can increase cortisol levels in the body, thereby making you feel stressed. The health benefits of intermittent fasting may quickly get negated by increased levels of stress. What's more, high levels of stress hormone has been linked with fat storage, making it opposed to weight loss.
- **Hair loss and irregular menstrual periods:** Intermittent fasting could make you lose hair or miss your period as a result of a severe calorie deficit. Due to reduced blood glucose levels associated with fasting, you are also likely to feel colder while fasting.
- **The breakfast saga:** It has been asserted and reiterated countless times that breakfast is the most vital food of the day, and there is a solid argument behind it. Having breakfast within one hour of waking from sleep is vital to health, as it helps to facilitate metabolism. Intermittent fasting protocols do not support or encourage having breakfast. The body goes into a catabolic state in the night hours. Therefore, it is crucial that you eat breakfast within an hour of waking up in order to avoid further catabolism. Having breakfast latest an hour after waking up promotes lean body fitness and reduces your chances of binge-eating later in the day. So not eating breakfast, contrary to what some intermittent fasting experts say, might be detrimental to your muscle content.
- **Development of acidity:** Research has proved that alkaline diets are the best diets to stay on. This is so because an alkaline food content can counter the acidic impacts of foods, and help your weight loss endeavor. Intermittent fasting keeps you away from this benefit. When you fast for a long period of time, your body might get into an acidic state. An acidic body is more likely to fall prey to disease conditions than an alkaline body. Certain headaches, such as migraines, may also result from body acidity.
- **Blood sugar levels:** While high blood sugar levels are detrimental to health, low levels of blood sugar are not good either. Regular diets can help regulate your blood sugar levels

naturally, a feat that intermittent fasting cannot achieve. Intermittent fasting can cause blood sugar levels to drop, thereby disrupting your body's regulatory process. In the long term, skipping meals can lead to general body weakness and lethargy.

- **Hormonal imbalance:** Intermittent fasting can cause hormonal imbalance by disrupting the body's normal diet patterns. People suffering from illnesses caused by hormonal imbalance can have their case worsened through engaging in intermittent fasting.

- **Diarrhea:** This is one of the common side effects felt by individuals who are just starting on intermittent fasting, especially if they have had a lot of carbohydrate-containing foods prior to fasting. Another potential cause of diarrhea in intermittent fasting is the drastic reduction in insulin, which is a signal to the kidneys to excrete more water. Diarrhea can be highly uncomfortable. A viable solution to this problem is to put a tablespoon of psyllium husk in a cup of water, let it stand for about ten minutes, and then drink it as a first meal in the morning. You may repeat this later on if you feel the need to do so. In addition, add a pinch of salt to your drinking water.

- **Anxiety and sleep deprivation:** Intermittent fasting leads to the production of the hormone Adrenaline, which may cause anxiety and insomnia. The hormone is typically a good hormone, helping us feel a boost in energy and keeping us alert. But the problem is, sometimes we need to be asleep. And this hormone can keep us awake at a time we seriously need to be in bed. The hormone can also cause to be jittery. Some individuals who have tried intermittent fasting have reported feeling like they consumed too much coffee in their early fasting days. People suffering from anxiety may begin to worry that fasting makes this condition worse, even though it may not. Why the jittering is worse is simply down to the fact that you produce more adrenaline during fasting. Because we are a species that adapt quickly to strange circumstances, we are often able to adjust to the higher than normal levels of adrenaline. Make sure you stick to a good bedtime routine.

- **Acid reflux:** It is yet unclear why some people experience acid reflux while fasting. However, it may be inferred that this side effect often happens in people who have a medical history of acid reflux. It seldom happens that a person who doesn't have a history of acid reflux would suddenly develop it for the first time while fasting. The good news is if you have acid reflux while fasting, then be sure that the condition would disappear once your body gets acclimatized to fasting. If you have a history of acid reflux, then ensure to take measures that would prevent the condition from resurfacing or becoming worse during fasting. Take anything from one to three tablespoons of lemon juice in your drinking water on the fasting day. You may also include the same amount of raw apple cider vinegar to your water throughout the day. Avoid substances that can make the condition worse or trigger it, such as broth, peppermint tea, and pickle juice.

- **Gout:** As is the case with acid reflux, it is not quite clear why some people develop gout while fasting. Also, it seldom happens that a person with no medical history of gout can suddenly come up with it all of a sudden during fasting. Endeavor to take cheery root extracts and include a tablespoon or two to your drinking water throughout the day. If you have a history of gout, then go slowly with intermittent fasting at first. Don't rush in. Be a little mild with the fasting and grow into it as time progresses.

- **Bad breath:** This is an example of a negative consequence that comes out of great things. When you lose weight, it is normal to have bad breath. This is called keto breath. Keto breath makes your tongue whitish and has an acetone taste because acetone is a substance produced during fat metabolism. Some people freak out when they experience tongue whitening, thinking they have some kind of bad infection. The truth is, your body is simply burning fat, and it will all go away soon enough. The solution to this condition is to take more water, use a tongue scraper, and brush your teeth more often than usual.

Like all things that have great benefits, intermittent fasting does not come without its shortfalls. These shortfalls range from mild symptoms, such as tongue whitening and bad breath, to more serious medical conditions, like gout, constipation, and insomnia. Intermittent fasting is not for everyone, sadly.

No matter how much you would like to shed some weight and keep a lean body if you have certain health conditions that are contraindicated to intermittent fasting, then it is highly recommended that you find other ways you achieve your weight loss and muscle building goals. If you don't have a full-blown health condition yet but have risk factors for one, then endeavor to check in with your caregiver for advice and recommendations before you venture into intermittent fasting. If you fail to do this, you may be doing your body a great injustice. What's more, you may actually end up harming your body and gaining much less than you gain from your intermittent fasting journey.

CONCLUSION

Intermittent fasting, as an eating pattern, is gaining further ground daily. The idea of fasting intermittently for a prolonged period of time is rooted in the notion that restricting your body's calorie consumption can lead to weight loss. Furthermore, muscle gain is possible during intermittent fasting as long as the right diets in their appropriate ratios are used to supported muscle gain efforts. The benefits of intermittent fasting, however, far surpass weight loss and mass muscle gain alone.

They include a myriad of health benefits, including improved cardiovascular health, reduced risks for developing certain chronic illnesses like Alzheimer's disease and cancer, increased insulin sensitivity and consequent improvement in blood sugar, and reduced risks of inflammation, among other benefits. More studies are being done in the area of the benefits of intermittent fasting, and the list of health benefits it offers is seemingly endless.

There are many intermittent fasting protocols to choose from – the 16/8 or the lean gains protocol, the 5:2 protocol or the fast diet, the eat-stop-diet protocol, and the warrior protocol. Each of these protocols has specific instructions and guidelines as to how dieters can and should fashion their feasting and fasting windows. The lean gains protocol states that a dieter should fast for 16 hours and eat in a 4-hour window every day. The fast diet proposes an entirely different plan, where a dieter can eat normally for 5 days and fast for any 2 non-consecutive days of the week. The way stop eat protocol is a rather flexible one, on which a dieter should fast for 24 consecutive hours once or twice in a week or two. In the warrior diet, a dieter can eat any amount of food in a 4-hour window but must fast for the next twenty hours. All of these protocols are fairly easy to understand and follow and have unique benefits and perks.

The flexibility and wealth of options regarding intermittent fasting protocols mean that you, the dieter, have an advantage in the intermittent fasting world. You can peruse the options available to you, assess them, and choose the one that suits best with your personal preferences and unique circumstances. While you may pick and choose as you see fit, the truth is, no matter what protocol you decide to start on, you'll be left with an incredible tool to lose weight, gain muscle, and improve your overall state of health.